mindful eating
on the go

books by Jan Chozen Bays

How to Train a Wild Elephant:
And Other Adventures in Mindfulness

Jizo Bodhisattva: Guardian of Children,
Travelers, and Other Voyagers

Mindful Eating: A Guide to Rediscovering
a Healthy and Joyful Relationship with Food
(also available as an audiobook)

Mindfulness on the Go: Simple Meditation
Practices You Can Do Anywhere

The Vow-Powered Life:
A Simple Method for Living with Purpose

also available

Mindfulness on the Go Cards: 52 Simple
Meditation Practices You Can Do Anywhere

mindful eating
on the go

practices for eating with awareness,
wherever you are

Jan Chozen Bays, MD

Shambhala
Boulder 2018

Shambhala Publications, Inc.
4720 Walnut Street
Boulder, Colorado 80301
www.shambhala.com

This book is a revised and abridged version of *Mindful Eating*
(Shambhala, 2017).

9 8 7 6 5 4 3 2 1

First Edition
Printed in the United States of America

♾ This edition is printed on acid-free paper that meets the American
National Standards Institute Z39.48 Standard.
♻ This book is printed on 30% postconsumer recycled paper.
For more information please visit www.shambhala.com.

Shambhala Publications is distributed worldwide by Penguin Random
House, Inc., and its subsidiaries.

Designed by Liz Quan

LIBRARY OF CONGRESS CATALOGING-IN-PUBLICATION DATA

Names: Bays, Jan Chozen.
Title: Mindful eating on the go: practices for eating with awareness, wher-
    ever you are / Jan Chozen Bays, MD.
Other titles: Mindful eating
Description: Boulder: Shambhala, 2018. | Compact version of: Mindful
    eating /Jan Chozen Bays.
Identifiers: LCCN 2018015779 | ISBN 9781611806335 (paperback)
Subjects: LCSH: Food habits—Psychological aspects. | Gastronomy. |
    Eating Disorders—Treatment. | Mindfulness-based cognitive therapy. |
Consciousness—Religious aspects—Buddhism. | Meditation—Therapeutic
    use. | BISAC: BODY, MIND & SPIRIT / Meditation. | SELF-HELP / Eating
    Disorders. | HEALTH & FITNESS / Healthy Living.
Classification: LCC TX357 .B455 2018 | DDC 641.01/3—dc23
LC record available at https://lccn.loc.gov/2018015779

dedication

May you discover the wisdom that resides
in your own body, heart, and mind.

May you enjoy good health and
continue the adventure of mindful eating
throughout your life, making many, many
interesting discoveries.

contents

mindful eating
on the go

introduction

Eating is one of the most pleasurable experiences we have in life.

Yet, somehow, for many of us, it has become a source of suffering. When people learned that I was writing the book *Mindful Eating*, they would often confess to some kind of difficulty with eating, ranging from "I eat when I'm anxious," to "I've had bulimia for ten years," to "Every time I sit down to eat, fear rises up in me."

I wrote this book to address an increasingly widespread and unnecessary form of suffering. You could call this an epidemic of disordered eating, but I prefer to think of the problem as an out-of-balance relationship with food. Researchers have found that Americans worry more about food and derive less pleasure from it than people in any other nation they surveyed. Our anxious minds have stolen something from our bodies and hearts. They have stolen our birthright to simply enjoy the innate pleasure and comfort of eating. Our resulting struggles with food can cause tremendous distress, guilt, shame, and depression.

One of the primary causes of this imbalance is a lack of an essential human nutrient: mindfulness. Mindfulness is the act of paying full, nonjudgmental attention to our moment-to-moment experience.

> **Mindful eating is deliberately paying attention to what is happening both inside yourself—in body, mind, and heart—and outside yourself, in your environment, while you eat. Mindful eating involves full awareness without criticism or judgment.**

The words "without criticism or judgment" are very important. Mindful eating is an adventure marked by curiosity, investigation, discovery, and an increasing sense of being liberated. Liberated from what? From the prison of rules, rigid control, guilt, and shame.

This little book is not about diets, exchanges, charts, or scales. Mindful eating is not dictated by an outside expert. It is directed by your inner experience, moment by moment. Your experience is unique. Therefore, you are the expert. Will you lose or gain weight if you bring mindfulness into cooking and eating? I don't know. What you could lose is the weight of the mind's unhappiness with eating and dissatisfaction with food. What you could gain is a simple joy with the food on your plate and an easy pleasure in eating. These are your birthrights as a human being.

People often tell me, "I would like to practice mindfulness, but my life is so busy that I don't have even fifteen minutes of extra time in my day." Mindfulness is not a chore, something you must squeeze into an already full schedule of working, raising children, and caring for a home. Mindfulness doesn't require extra time. It simply asks us to remember to bring a quality of purposeful awareness to the ordinary activities of the life we are already living.

That sounds easy, but remembering is actually the hardest part of being mindful. Even though I've been practicing and teaching mindful eating for more than thirty years, I still forget. One mindful eating exercise that always makes me laugh is called "One Bite at a Time, or Put Down That Utensil!" (page 121). It's one of my favorite mindful eating practices, and I've done it thousands of times, but I still catch my mind wandering off and my hand sneaking in to put a second bite into my mouth before the first one is swallowed.

I'm often asked about how I decided to write a book about mindful eating. It happened when I became aware of the epidemic of obesity in children and the prediction that children born in this decade would live shorter lives than their parents due to obesity-related complications, including type 2 diabetes and liver damage.

When I reviewed the approaches we've tried in the past to help bring natural balance back into eating, I realized that conventional methods aren't working. They are all flawed, as well as totally unsuitable for children. I felt we needed a fresh approach, a treatment that would be inexpensive or free, accessible to people of all ages and economic levels, and something parents could learn and teach to their children. I wanted to find a treatment with positive side effects, transferring benefit to other aspects of life, and most important, an approach that was fun. At this point, two separate streams in my life came together—my work as a pediatrician and my work as a Zen teacher. I realized that mindful eating might be the "treatment" I'd been looking for.

Mindful eating is fun! No matter what our age or condition, we all have to eat and drink, which gives us at least three to six opportunities a day to bring the power of mindfulness into our lives. You don't have to go to a weeklong silent retreat or live at a monastery. This adventure is always available and begins each time we raise a glass or fork. No passports or airline reservations needed.

Many years ago, when I did my first weeklong silent Zen retreat, I carefully followed the instructions to be fully aware of every breath, every movement, and every passing sensation. As I was eating a silent meal, I paid careful attention to the flavors and changing textures in my mouth, the movements of my tongue, and the phenomenon of swallowing. I traced the path of the food down my throat, into my stomach, out into my blood stream and into my cells, down to my toes. Suddenly, I was overwhelmed by the continuous experience of coming into union with the food. I realized, "Oh, this is communion! This is what my childhood church was trying to tell me all along!" I have continued to explore mindful eating for three decades, teaching it to many Zen students and health professionals.

The food we eat contains the life force of innumerable creatures, brought to us that we might have life and have it more abundantly. When something opens the door between our life and the mystery that is present—yet often hidden—in every moment of our life, we are fed from the source of deepest truth. If this happens when we are eating, physical food becomes spiritual food.

diets don't work

In affluent countries, our usual ways of dealing with problems are these: imprison, attack, or apply science and technology. Dieting involves putting certain foods in prison. You can eat all you want of this food, but that other food you have to shut out of your life and never touch again! If dieting worked, there would be one or two diet books, and they would work for everyone. People who undertake any diet will typically lose eight to twelve pounds and then regain that weight plus more within two years. In fact, research on dieting shows that if your goal is to gain weight, develop an eating disorder, and slow down your metabolism, then you should go on a diet, go off that diet, go back on a new diet, and go off again. Repeat. This is called "yo-yoing."

The basic problem with dieting is that it trains people to turn to and rely on *external sources of authority*: diet gurus, calorie counting, exchanges, packaged or liquid meals, and the latest celebrity-endorsed diet plan. Mindful eating returns you to *internal sources of authority*: your body, your heart, and your mind. These are your own trustworthy sources of wisdom and compassion. Plus, they are free and always available!

Professionals who take our mindful eating trainings often say, "We are tired of handing out diet sheets to patients, when they know and we know that they won't follow them. It's an exercise in futility. Mindful eating is the missing piece!"

Other solutions our culture has tried in the past involve attacking our body fat or our digestive system. Liposuction can remove some fat cells, but if we continue consuming extra calories, fat cells in other locations will grow larger. The problem is not in our fat cells, which are just trying to do their job of storing extra calories as insurance against times of famine—famine that never arrives.

We've invented bariatric surgery to rearrange our digestive system so that our stomachs are much smaller or the part of our small intestine that actually absorbs nutrients is diverted, so what we eat passes through and doesn't actually nourish our bodies. After bariatric surgery only one in ten people attain their target weight, and up to a third eventually gain weight back. When food can no longer be used to relieve distress, some people develop transfer addiction to alcohol, opiates, gambling, shopping, or sex. This occurs in about 25 percent of patients. The problem is not in our digestive system, which is just trying to do its job—digest and absorb nutrients so we will be healthy.

We've also applied technology. There are many apps that claim to promote weight loss, slower eating, or even mindful eating. With apps, of course, we are back to an outside source of authority telling us how to eat. You can spend forty dollars on a fork that buzzes when it's OK to take another bite, four hundred dollars for a dental appliance that limits the space in your mouth so you must take smaller bites, or ten thousand dollars for a tube that pumps food out of your stomach and into the toilet. I'm not kidding. The problem is not in our forks or spoons, our mouths or stomachs, which all continually work to support us in nourishing ourselves.

Research shows there is something that does work to help us enjoy eating and change our eating habits: it's mindful eating, specifically learning to pay attention to what we eat and slowing down a bit.

mindful eating is not about learning something new

Mindful eating is about rediscovering your innate ability to eat in a healthy way. This was an ability you had in childhood that was subverted by many influences: your parents' anxiety ("Don't eat that candy! You'll get fat!"); soda in vending machines at school; television ads that encourage you to eat cereal while playing video games; bullying in school; and anorexic models in clothing ads.

You might think that the title *Mindful Eating on the Go* is at odds with the practice of mindful eating, which does include learning ways to slow down and savor your food. It's true that research shows that when people are taught to slow down their eating and to pay greater attention to what they are eating, they will eat more appropriate foods and in healthier quantities. However, our lives are busy, and at times we must eat quickly—for example, when a lunch break is shortened by a client, customer, or urgent call. We can still practice mindful eating as we take the first few bites of food or sips of liquid.

Mindful Eating on the Go is designed to go with you. You can tuck it in your pocket or desk drawer and read one exercise in just a few minutes. It can help remind you to explore the many opportunities you have each day to stop briefly and enter a more vivid experience of your life, to come into presence. Life quickly passes by, and our opportunity to be awake and experience it fully will too soon be lost.

When mindful eating is ignored, it causes pervasive and unnecessary suffering. When mindfulness is applied to eating, a world of discovery and delight opens. This is a world that has been hidden, quite literally, beneath our noses.

It is my sincere wish that this little book will help you to open yourself to the joy and delight, the richness and splendor, of the simple acts of eating and drinking, so that you can find true, deep, and lasting satisfaction with food and enjoy eating throughout your life.

how to use this book

There are many ways to use this book. It contains twenty-three exercises to help bring mindfulness into your relationship to food. You can move through them from the beginning, doing one exercise each week for twenty-three weeks.

You can begin with the exercises on the Nine Hungers, followed by "Putting It All Together: Who's Hungry in There?" This will help you become acquainted with each aspect of hunger and learn to assess them all quickly before you eat and also before deciding about second helpings.

When you learn to check in with the Nine Hungers, your relationship with food and eating will be transformed. You will learn to "hear" and trust the wisdom of your closest companion, your body. It will become your ally. When we eat mindfully, our eating is transformed from a source of anxiety and shame into a source of refreshment, self-confidence, and happiness.

You can also customize your exploration, picking an exercise to try for one day that fits your own needs or whims. However, practicing the same exercise every day for a whole week provides a longer interval for discoveries and insights to arise. It also contains the advantage of more coherent practice time, which can help you to stabilize the new practice and integrate it into your routine.

You also may find it helpful to use the audio recordings for a number of the exercises described in the book. They are listed on pages 156–57 and are available at www.shambhala.com/mindfuleating. On the website you'll also find a link to download images as visual reminders to help you practice the various mindfulness exercises in this book.

For each exercise there is a description of "The Exercise" and some ideas about "Reminding Yourself" to do it throughout the day and week. Next, we discuss some of the "Discoveries" that individuals have made about that exercise or that have been revealed by scientific or medical research. The section ends with "Deeper Lessons" that can be uncovered as you continue the practice. For some of the Nine Hungers I've included ways to feed that hunger without using food. Each exercise is like a window, giving us a glimpse of what an awakened life might be like. A few "Final Words" sum up the exercise and inspire you to continue letting it unfold.

Once you've worked through the book, the Summary Tips section on pages 153–155 might be a helpful way to quickly remind yourself of some of the most important mindful eating principles and practices.

This is a book to carry with you, to bring investigation, discovery, and enjoyment into eating. It might seem that I am giving this lovely practice to you, but as a small child, you knew how to eat effortlessly, happily, and mindfully. Thus, it is a gift you already have, one that you can simply retrieve from its hiding place, dust off, and give back to yourself.

part one

the nine aspects of hunger

The *Nine Hungers* is shorthand for the nine different aspects of what we lump together and call "hunger." Why are the nine aspects of hunger important? Hunger is a multisensory experience. Our eyes, our nose, our mouth, our stomach, our cells, our heart, and even our mind can all send us signals that we interpret as hunger. We are easily confused about who in there—what part of us—is hungry. Exploring each aspect separately can help us understand which kind of hunger is calling to us and thus make better decisions about eating.

Here's an example of the benefits of familiarity with the Nine Hungers. A woman who decided to have bariatric surgery told me that she was grateful for the mindful eating classes she had taken in the two years beforehand. After the operation she attended a support group at the hospital. Many women were distressed and complained, "I thought the surgery would take away my hunger. But I'm still hungry!" My student said that the others in the support group didn't realize that stomach hunger had been reduced by the surgery, but eye hunger, ear hunger, nose hunger, mouth hunger, and especially heart hunger were still clamoring, "I'm hungry, let's eat!"

Heart hunger is particularly important. Eating to relieve distress in our heart only provides temporary relief. We have to learn emotional intelligence, recognizing which emotion has triggered the desire to eat and then addressing that emotion directly. When heart hunger is not recognized, people can try to use food to soothe their distress, but soon they find that the inner critic is attacking them for eating inappropriately. The additional anxiety created by the inner critic can catalyze a vicious cycle: feel badly > eat > feel worse because you ate > eat more > and so on, around and around. Mindful eating helps us step back and ask, what emotion did I feel just before I felt compelled to eat? Once we can identify the emotion, we can apply a better remedy than compulsive eating. If you're lonely, call a friend or cuddle your dog. If you're tired and irritable, take a nap. Or renew yourself by meditating or going for a walk outside, taking deep breaths of fresh air.

I think you will enjoy exploring the nine aspects of hunger and learn that you can rely on them to help you make wise decisions about eating. Let's begin!

1

eye hunger

the exercise

For one week, be conscious of the things that appeal to your eye hunger. Notice photos in magazines, on menus, in the supermarket, online, and on billboards. When you sit down to eat (you do sit down to eat, don't you?) notice what foods appeal to your eyes. Purposely look at what you are eating. Notice if your eating experience changes when you don't look at your food. If you prepare your own meals, take extra care this week to consider eye appeal.

reminding yourself

Post a picture of an eye or put a note saying "eye hunger" in your lunch box or where you usually eat.

Buy a food magazine and keep it someplace where you'll see it each day. Maybe on your bedside table. Glance through a few pages each day this week, noting what appeals to your eyes and makes you hungry.

discoveries

You've just finished dinner at a nice restaurant and you feel completely full—well, maybe a bit overfull.

Friendly server: "Would you like some dessert?"

You: "No, I'm really full and quite satisfied. It was delicious, but I couldn't eat another bite. Can we put the rest in a doggie bag?"

Server (sensing some hesitation): "Sure, I'll get you a box, but how about I just show you the dessert tray?"

Your mind: "It can't hurt."

So the server brings the dessert tray: New York cheesecake with raspberry sauce, chocolate mousse with a swirl of whipped cream, hot apple pie with caramel sauce, and a lemon tart with a chocolate truffle on top.

Your eyes: "We could eat one of those!"

Your mouth: "Of course we can!"

The old saying "Your eyes are bigger than your stomach" comes true when your stomach is full but your eyes make the decision to eat more.

Our eyes have a great deal of power in deciding what to eat and how much to eat. This may be because the ability for hunter-gatherers to forage for edible and energy-rich plants and animals was essential to human survival during the majority of our evolution, when food was scarce. Our brains require 25 percent of our total energy intake, so it benefits them to help us find foods with a high-calorie content.

Scientists question whether the epidemic of obesity has been expanded by the overabundance of food in supermarkets and restaurants, the popularity of cooking shows that glamorize food, and especially the pervasive images of food on social media (called "food pornography"). Most of these images show food high in calories and fat. In 2014 and 2015 food was the second most frequently searched category on the internet. (Pornography was first.) A recent survey revealed that 63 percent of thirteen- to thirty-two-year-olds have posted a photo of food or drink that they (or someone else) were having on social media. There are now more than fifty-four million pictures of food just on Instagram. Some chefs have banned diners from taking photos of their food, while others encourage it as free publicity and may even provide a camera stand.

Pictures of food may make us hungry for high-calorie foods, but such images can also pull us away from paying full attention to the flavors and textures of the food we are actually eating. Full attention is the source of satisfaction. Virtual food does not satisfy the mouth, stomach, body, or heart.

Few foods are colored blue, perhaps because humans are naturally wary of food that might be moldy. If you dye food odd colors, people react in interesting ways. In one experiment, the lights in a test restaurant were kept dim to disguise the actual colors of the food. When the lights were turned up and the diners saw that the steak was dyed blue, the chips green, and the peas red, many complained of feeling ill. In another study, when a strawberry drink was colored green, 27 percent of tasters described its flavor as lime.

Research shows that people generally decide how much food they will eat based upon feedback from the eyes. Given a large box of free but stale popcorn, they will dip in twenty-one more times and eat 173 more calories than those given a medium-size bucket. We serve ourselves more food if we are offered a large plate or bowl, because the same portion size looks like less food on a large plate. In America, people often decide to stop eating when they see that the plate is empty or the TV show is over, whereas in France people are more likely to stop eating when the food has "lost its appeal."

Advertisers know about eye hunger. They hire photographers whose specialty is photographing food to maximize its appeal to the eye. Magazines such as *Gourmet* and *Women's Day* are filled with delicious pictures that make you want to get out the mixing bowls and preheat the oven. When you go to a movie, it's hard not to head to the concession stand when a giant box of hot buttered popcorn or a six-foot candy bar appears on the screen.

deeper lessons

If you wish to eat less, your eyes can help you. Use smaller plates, bowls, and utensils to take advantage of the size illusion. You can help prevent eye hunger from taking over by serving yourself in a different location from where you eat. Keep serving bowls out of sight. Out of sight, out of mind is true. If we stop feeding desire with sights and thoughts of what we desire, the desire will lose its power. If your eyes demand, "That looks yummy; let's eat some," pause to consult your stomach to see if it is already full, and ask your body whether this additional food will support the health of your cells and organs.

There are ways to nourish yourself through your eyes without using food. Notice the shape and color of your empty plate. Serve yourself and then, before you eat, look at the food as if it were a work of art—become aware of the different colors, shapes, and surface textures.

The eyes enjoy beauty. Take a few minutes several times a day to pause and really look at things in your environment—a bright flower, a softly moving shadow, the colors and shapes of the things on your desk, the sparkly bits in the pavement as you walk.

FINAL WORDS

If eye hunger takes over, we may eat inappropriate kinds and amounts of food. Remember that beauty is all around you, and you can feed on it with your eyes. Just stop and really look!

touch hunger

the exercise

Become aware of the touch sensations as you eat, including textures such as smooth, crunchy, creamy, lumpy, soft, hard, and crisp. For at least one meal, put away utensils and try eating just with your hands. (You may need napkins and a finger bowl of warm water at hand.)

reminding yourself

Post a picture of fingers and a tongue or a note saying "touch hunger" near where you usually eat. Make a reservation at a restaurant where you eat with your fingers.

discoveries

There are two categories of touch hunger: the sensations on your tongue and the sensations of your fingers when you eat with your hands.

Mouthfeel is a term for the sensations that food or drink create in your mouth and throat. Diners most often send dishes back to the kitchen for issues of texture, not taste (think about limp french fries or tough meat). Mouthfeel has become very important in the wine industry, which has a wonderful vocabulary to describe attributes of wine. A "softer, rounder, broader, and fatter" mouthfeel is currently popular among wine drinkers, and the industry has a variety of methods and additives to produce this effect, including adding glycerol or certain yeast strains or aging wine with toasted oak chips. Also, wine makers have found that when the viscosity of wine is increased, we perceive it to be sweeter. The Japanese lead the world in awareness of mouthfeel, with more than four hundred terms for different aspects, compared with about seventy-five in English.

Every culture has foods that can be eaten politely with your hands. In the United States these include many snack or fast foods, crackers and cheese, chips and dip, fried chicken, hamburgers, french fries, tacos, Buffalo wings, pizza, toast, and cookies. It does not include rice and curry, cornmeal mush with peanut sauce, or bread with fish sauce. Yet in India, Malawi, and Ethiopia, respectively, those foods are always eaten with the fingers.

In many countries people eat only with their hands. They say that using utensils is like attacking the food with metal weapons. They are emphatic that eating with their hands is a much more mindful and intimate experience, that you can better regulate the amount you eat, and that it makes the food taste better. There are rules: wash your hands before and after eating and use your right hand only (the left is reserved for personal hygiene). Usually you pick up a small ball of rice or flat bread and then dip it in a vegetable or meat sauce before popping it into your mouth.

Often people sit around a table with serving dishes placed in the center. Someone may put a delicious morsel on another person's plate. This creates a feeling of warmth and intimacy, as people share both food and conversation. Ethiopian restaurants have always encouraged people to eat in this traditional style, and some Indian restaurants in large cities are now also serving food with utensils only by request.

If you are adventurous, why don't you try eating an entire meal with your hands? This may seem strange at first. (Soup can be eaten with a spoon or drunk from the bowl.) If you don't want to do this at home, go to an Indian, Middle Eastern, or Ethiopian restaurant and ask the waiter for advice on how to eat without utensils. See for yourself if it slows you down or adds attentiveness or sensual pleasure to your meal.

Babies enjoy feeding themselves with their hands, although their parents may need to clean up food in the baby's hair, down their shirtfront, and on the floor. New research shows that if they are allowed to eat with their hands, babies eat more appropriate amounts and kinds of foods, and are less likely to become obese. It is a way they can learn self-regulation, or what I call the "appestat" (appetite thermostat), the inner signal that tells you when to stop eating. When adults push a certain food out of anxiety or stuff "one last bite" into a resisting mouth in order to finish the jar or bowl of food, they are teaching the child to override the wisdom of their own body's feedback signals about how much is enough.

deeper lessons

Human beings thrive when they are touched. Studies show that touch deprivation, also called "skin hunger," can lead to a variety of health and psychological problems, and that massage is therapeutic for many different conditions. Massage can help lower high blood pressure, improve lung function in children with asthma, increase mobility in people with Parkinson's, lower blood sugar in people with diabetes, and reduce anxiety, depression, and pain. If one medicine had this many positive effects, it would be called a "wonder drug." These effects seem to be mediated by reduction in the stress hormone cortisol and increased secretion of feel-good hormones like dopamine, serotonin, and oxytocin.

Touch is not the sense we usually focus on while we are eating; smell and taste are foremost in our awareness. However, the touch sensation we call "texture" can be very important. Think of your dismay when you bite into a soggy potato chip. Becoming mindful of touch and texture sensations can improve your experience of eating. Enjoy the creaminess of chocolate as it melts on your tongue, the spongy texture of whipped cream, and the crunch of nuts or raw carrots.

With our modern emphasis on cleanliness, eating with our hands may seem strange, messy, or unsanitary at first. Ayurvedic (traditional Indian) medicine teaches that when food is picked up with the fingers, certain nutrients are actually absorbed through the skin, causing digestive hormones to be released. This is said to lead to feeling satisfied with less food. Eating with the hands tends to slow down the speed of eating, which does help people eat less.

When you eat with awareness of touch, you widen your awareness to include not just your hands but also the exquisite touch sensitivity of your lips and tongue. Your tongue can detect tiny particles stuck in your teeth and returns to them again and again until it is able to pry them out. Try savoring a small piece of chocolate as it dissolves in your mouth. If you try a second or third piece, what happens to the flavor or pleasure of the experience?

There are ways to nourish yourself through your sense of touch without using food. Hug yourself tenderly. Give a sore place in your body a gentle massage. Take a warm shower or leisurely bath and open your senses to the touch of the water.

FINAL WORDS

Being mindful of touch and texture sensations as you eat can bring more pleasure and satisfaction to eating.

3

ear hunger

the exercise

Try preparing and eating a meal or snack in silence. As you eat, pay special attention to all the sounds that come to your ears. For example, listen to the many sounds involved just in making toast: the toaster button being pushed down, the toast popping up, the knife cutting butter, the crunch as you first bite in, and the sounds inside your head of chewing and swallowing.

When you are eating with others, at a table or in a cafeteria or restaurant, take a few minutes to just listen to the "music" of eating, as if you were a modern composer taking in ideas for a new avant-garde symphony. What do you hear? Silverware on china? Chairs scraping? The murmur of conversation at a nearby table? A cell phone ringing? It might be lovely or amusing!

reminding yourself

Post a picture of an ear or put a note saying "ear hunger" in your lunch box or near where you eat.

discoveries

We seldom notice the sounds of eating, but it turns out that the sounds our ears hear as we eat are surprisingly critical to our enjoyment of eating. There are some foods we expect to make noise when we eat them, like raw carrots or potato chips, and some foods we expect to be quiet, like pudding or ice cream.

Dr. Charles Spence of Oxford University is a specialist in multisensory or cross-modal aspects of perception. He was given the Ig Nobel Prize, for unusual imaginative research that makes people laugh and then think, for a study showing that changing the pitch and volume of the "crunch" of a potato chip altered people's perception of how crisp and fresh it was. No crunch or the wrong pitch to the crunch, and we think it might be soggy or stale. Likewise, if we're eating creamy pudding and suddenly hear a crunch in our mouth, we worry about a contaminant or whether we've just lost a filling from a tooth.

Our strong preference for foods involving crunchy, crispy, or crackling sounds may arise from the implication that the food is fresh. A Cheetos ad proclaimed, "The cheese that goes crunch!" The Frito-Lay company claimed that research proved that Doritos produced the loudest crack.

Part of our pleasure in eating comes from what we hear. When people are blindfolded and white noise is piped into their earphones, the higher the volume, the less salty or sweet they rate the food they are eating. Loud ambient noise may explain why the food served on airplanes and to astronauts must be heavily seasoned to be enjoyed.

Some restaurants are quite noisy, with music played at decibels that are uncomfortable and make talking to your friends an exercise in reading lips. This may be a deliberate ploy. People eat more food (and drink more alcohol more quickly) when noise levels are higher and they cannot hear the sounds of their own eating and drinking. Loud music forces people to talk louder. It creates an atmosphere that makes (some) people feel excited and energized. More expensive restaurants tend to be quieter. They expect guests to relax and spend more time eating—and to tip better.

deeper lessons

Pets often come running when they hear the sound of a can opener. We are also creatures of conditioning. Are there sounds that make you hungry? Popping popcorn? Bacon sizzling? A bag of chips being torn open? The freezer door being opened? A person describing a delicious dinner they've eaten?

Ear hunger includes hunger that arises when we hear food or drink described. In one experiment a waiter announced a wine as coming from either a new winery in California or a new winery in North Dakota. The wine was the same; only the name of the state was changed on the label. Diners rated the "California wine" as better tasting than the "Dakota wine" and were willing to pay more money for it. What the ears hear can create expectations that interfere with our ability to be fully aware and appreciate the flavors we taste.

There are ways to nourish yourself through your ears without using food. There is a lovely meditation on sound. Sit quietly, eyes partly or completely closed, and open your ears to sound. Refrain from naming or thinking about the sounds. Listen as though listening to strange and interesting music from an alien planet. Listen for the obvious and then the subtler sounds. Can you hear anything that sounds like percussion? Listen for high notes and bass notes. Listen between the sounds—is there actually silence there?

If you are feeling harried or anxious, coming to a full stop and then opening your ears and *just listening* for a minute or two is an effective way to let go of thoughts, "reset" yourself, and then continue on in a better state of mind.

FINAL WORDS

When we open our ears, there is music everywhere! We are always smack in the middle of a concert—it's just being played on unusual instruments.

nose hunger

the exercise

Each time you have something to eat or drink, pause and inhale its aromas. If you aren't in polite company, you can bend down to be close to the food or lift the bowl or plate up to your nose. Close your eyes and sniff, then move away to refresh your nose, and sniff again. How would you describe what you smell?

reminding yourself

Post pictures of a nose inhaling aromas or put a note saying "nose hunger" in your lunch box or wherever you eat.

discoveries

When we say, "This tastes good," what we are actually describing is primarily the smell. Our tongues are able to taste only about five flavors: sweet, salty, sour, bitter, and umami (a savory or meaty taste). Everything else we call "taste" is actually aroma.

We don't completely appreciate our sense of smell until we lose it—for example, when we have a cold. If you love to eat, this loss can be very distressing. When we can't smell food, we perceive it as having almost no taste. Without smell all the subtlety of flavor is lost. Food becomes something you have to eat because your body needs fuel. You might as well save money and time by eating dog kibble.

When you lose your ability to smell, it's interesting to pay attention to what you *are* able to detect, which is just the tongue's five basic flavors. The only other characteristic that you notice is the textures of different foods, soft or crunchy. Just those five flavors and a few textures are not enough to interest us.

Merchants are very aware of nose hunger, and they count on it to entice you. Think of the smells of a bakery, a coffee shop, a fast-food hut, or a cinnamon bun stand that pipes an almost irresistible aroma all over the mall. The right smells will make us eat more. When researchers impregnated plastic bowls with the artificial odor of cinnamon and raisin, people ate more plain oatmeal than when the bowls were scented with a discordant scent, macaroni and cheese.

I can't eat chocolate anymore, but when I serve, say, chocolate truffles, I'll hold one, inhale deeply, and just enjoy the aroma. It's almost as good as eating it.

deeper lessons

The cells that respond to smells in the back of our nose are just two synapses away from the processing centers for emotion and memories in our primitive brain, so odors can evoke powerful conditioned responses such as desire and aversion. These unconscious responses can occur even when we are not aware of detecting an odor. People who lose their sense of smell permanently can become depressed. They lose their previous enjoyment of food or become anxious that they will not smell smoke from a fire or detect their own body odor, or might eat spoiled food. Although our tongues are able to register only a few taste sensations, we can distinguish several thousand odors. Our noses can detect as little as one molecule of some substances. Research shows that women have more sensitive noses than men. Women who wear perfume to attract men are probably wasting effort and money. The fragrances men pick as favorites are related to food—the smell of baking bread, vanilla, and grilling meat.

There are ways to nourish yourself through your nose, without eating food. Try a walking meditation, paying special attention to smells. If you are inside your home, try sniffing various products: soaps, cleaning powder, lotions, cosmetics. You can open spice jars and sample the different scents. Could you describe what you detect? Is there a spice scent that makes you feel more relaxed and calm? One that makes you feel more excited or energetic? Are there spices whose smell brings back memories?

FINAL WORDS

If you become conscious of the fragrance of food, it will enrich your experience of eating. If you become more aware of the various fragrances in your world, it will enrich the experience of this life you are living.

5

mouth hunger

the exercise

Before you eat, with the food in front of you, pause. Look at the food and become aware of the mouth's desire for food. Rate the mouth's hunger on a scale of zero (no mouth hunger) to ten (my mouth is ready to consume anything).

During the meal, pause every five minutes to assess mouth hunger. Does it change?

It is easier to keep track of mouth hunger if you are not doing anything else during the meal, such as talking, reading, or watching TV.

If you wish to expand your awareness of mouth hunger, notice it during the day. How does the mouth signal you, "Please put something in here"? What are the sensations of mouth hunger? See if you can ask the mouth what it wants and why. Does it want something salty, sweet, sour, crunchy, or creamy? Or are you actually thirsty?

reminding yourself

Post a picture of a mouth or a note saying "mouth hunger" in your lunch box or in the places you usually eat.

discoveries

The mouth loves sensations. Changing sensations. It might be happy with salty tortilla chips, but soon it becomes bored and demands salsa or a creamy dip to accompany them. Ask your mouth if it has had enough taste sensations today. I suspect it will say, "Why no, do you have something different or interesting for me to taste?" I call the mouth the "insatiable cavern of desire." When you are completely full, even overfull, and the server brings the dessert tray, both the eyes and mouth yell, "Yes, we can eat that!" Food manufacturers know the tastes and textures the mouth enjoys. They combine them all in foods such as salted caramel ice cream with nuts—sweet, salty, creamy, and crunchy. Food manufacturers know how to appeal to the mouth through what the eyes read. Just today on the grocery shelf I noticed Crunchy Flamin' Hot Cheetos! (with a picture of flames coming out of a chip), Cheese Explosion Doritos, Ghirardelli Intense Dark Raspberry Radiance chocolate bar, and Kellogg's Krave Double Chocolate breakfast cereal (with almost as much sugar as the candy bar).

Let's say that you've just sat down to enjoy a bowl of pasta with your favorite sauce. The first bite tastes so delicious! So does the second bite. You comment on the seasoning, and then begin a conversation with your friend about the best restaurants you have eaten in and the most delicious pasta dishes you've had. Suddenly you look down and see that the plate is empty. What happened to that wonderful pasta? After a few bites you didn't taste it, because you were busy talking. Instead of eating the food before you in *this* moment, *this* mouthful, you were thinking about memories of food from the past. The mouth's hunger has not been satisfied. The mouth asks for a second helping. It's still hungry. If you talk or watch TV while eating this second helping, you might feel oddly unsatisfied once again and need a third helping.

This is mindless eating. The mouth often tempts us into mindless eating. We all do it. We can all learn to change it. Even a small change, a few minutes of mindful eating each day, can offer a different way of experiencing the world around and within us.

By the time we have a third helping, the stomach is groaning. The mouth, however, could still be demanding more tastes. If you had been able to eat in silence, undistracted, with the "mind in the mouth," one helping might have been just enough. The key to satisfying mouth hunger is to be present, placing the focus of our mind in our mouth and opening our awareness to all the textures, movements, smells, sounds, and taste sensations of eating and drinking.

deeper lessons

One brand of chips used to advertise a "party in the mouth." To truly experience a party in the mouth, we don't need stronger flavoring. We need the presence of awareness. To satisfy the mouth's hunger for sensation, it isn't enough to put food into the mouth, chew it, and swallow it. If we want to feel satisfied as we eat, the mind has to be aware of what is occurring in the mouth. If we are distracted, we could be eating newspaper with sauce. If we are present and curious, even food that isn't our favorite can be surprisingly interesting.

Research shows that if people are trained to pay attention to what they are eating, they eat more appropriate kinds and quantities of food. As one man exclaimed during a mindful eating workshop, "Eating is the most pleasurable experience (besides sex) that I have, and I can have it several times a day. It's so self-defeating not to pay attention to it!" Yes.

Satisfaction and fullness are different experiences. Fullness is a physical sensation, a sensation of stretch and pressure in the abdomen. Satisfaction is an emotional experience, the experience of ease and calm. It does not depend upon quantity of food. A woman told me that she had lost thirty pounds in the year after attending a mindful eating workshop. How did she do it? She began to ponder the question, why do I eat? The answer that came was, to feel at peace. Therefore, she resolved to eat only until she felt peaceful inside. No special diet, nothing forced, just slowing down her eating so she could attend to internal sensations of agitation and notice when they changed into sensations of peace. Then stop.

We are all busy. Sometimes we have to eat quickly. But we can all take time to "feed the mouth" by really savoring the first few bites of food or the first few sips of a drink. The pleasure and satisfaction this brings may entice you to devote a little more time to eating with awareness.

FINAL WORDS

If you want to have a party in the mouth, the mind has to be invited.

stomach hunger

the exercise

Become aware of sensations coming from the area you call "my stomach" or "my gut." Before eating, bring your attention to your abdomen and ask your stomach how full it is: empty, a quarter full, half full, three-quarters full, full, or overfull? Then ask your stomach, "How much food would you be comfortable handling right now? One cup? Two cups? Three cups? Four cups? More?"

Repeat these questions halfway through the meal, and again at the end.

What can your stomach tell you about hunger and fullness?

reminding yourself

Post simple images of a stomach or a note saying "ask my stomach" in various places, including where you eat.

discoveries

Many of the signals that we identify as hunger come from our stomach. It growls or gurgles, cramps or gnaws, and tells us, "I'm uncomfortably empty!" It's embarrassing to admit this, since I'm a physician, but I didn't realize until I'd been doing mindful eating for years that the stomach does not taste food. The stomach has no taste buds! We might think, "My stomach is really going to like the taste of this food," but the stomach doesn't care.

What our stomach does care about is volume, which means how stretched it is. When we chronically overeat, we lose our ability to sense those signals of fullness. The stomach has to do a lot of work—sometimes hours of work—with what we send down to it. In mindful eating, we get back in touch with our stomach and treat it kindly. When people begin to eat mindfully, they often complain that when they ask their stomach these questions about fullness and volume, they aren't receiving a reply. However, if they keep asking, after a day or two, they begin to get, or maybe feel, an answer. This is exciting! It's the first step in a shift from looking to external sources of expertise about eating—diet books, TV gurus, movie stars—to the internal sources of wisdom in our own body, heart, and mind.

Some people discover that they are sitting down to eat a complete meal even when the signals from their stomach say that it is already full. They are eating just because the clock says noon or 6:00 P.M. Researchers from Columbia University showed that overweight people have a much greater tendency to ignore the signals from their stomachs and be influenced by external factors such as how attractively the food is presented or even what time they think it is. If a clock is manipulated to read noon when it is actually ten o'clock, they will eat a full lunch. People of average weight will not, because they are attuned to internal, not external, signals to tell them when they are hungry and when they are full.

Studies show that three-year-olds who are given a huge helping of macaroni and cheese will eat just enough and then stop. Five-year-olds, however, will make a valiant effort to eat it all. Their natural appestat has been shanghaied by adult pressure to "clean your plate" and "think of the starving children in Africa/China/India."

Knowing when we are full is a skill we all had in infancy and early childhood, but years of overeating can override the signals that our internal organs are constantly sending us. This is great news. We are not trying to invent something, just to relearn it.

deeper lessons

The people of Okinawa are among the world's longest lived. They have a saying, *hara no hachi bu*, which means to eat until you are four-fifths full (literally, eight parts out of ten). The first four parts support your good health, but if you eat that last fifth, it will support your doctor. People who learn to check in with their stomach several times during a meal almost always find that they feel quite satisfied with less food than they are accustomed to eating—when the eyes and mouth were conspiring to make decisions about portion size and whether to take seconds, ignoring the stomach.

One man in a mindful eating workshop exclaimed, "I've been so unkind to my stomach! From now on, I'm going to respect what it tells me." We expect our bodies to work perfectly, and when they don't, we become cranky. "I used to be able to eat a quarter-pound steak," "I used to be able to eat really spicy food," "Why do I get heartburn if I drink soda?" We feel that something is wrong with us if we cannot do, or eat, like we did ten years ago.

Nothing thrives under a bombardment of irritation and annoyance. Our bodies, like everything else, are constantly changing. If we are able to acknowledge that flux, and adjust to it, we will be much happier. When we listen to what our stomach tells us, give it only the appropriate amounts and kinds of food, and let it rest between meals, it and we will be much happier. We have only one body for this lifetime. It works hard to take care of us, day and night, and we need to take good care of it in return.

There is a simple way to send the nourishment of loving-kindness to your stomach. It is derived from Qigong, the ancient Chinese exercises for balancing the body's energy and promoting relaxation and health. Place your hand on your belly and gently rub in a circle, making twenty-four gradually larger circles. Then reverse direction and make twenty-four gradually smaller circles. When you finish, let your hand rest softly on your belly for a minute.

FINAL WORDS

Become friends with your stomach. Ask it for advice and then follow it. It can help guide you to better health.

7

cellular or body hunger

the exercise

Several times during the day bring your awareness to your body, particularly the lower half. Ask your cells or your entire body, "What would be good for you to eat or drink now?"

Try a walk through a grocery store when you are not hungry. Walk slowly around the outer aisles (generally where nonprocessed, real foods are located) and ask your body as you pass different foods and drinks, "What would be nourishing for you now?"

reminding yourself

Post a picture of a body or a note saying "cellular hunger" in places you usually eat. You also might set an alarm to ring a few times a day at random intervals. When it rings, pause briefly and ask your body the same question, "What would be nourishing for you now?"

discoveries

When we were infants, we were tuned in to the signals from our body that told us when to eat and when to stop. Given a choice, we had an instinctive awareness of which foods and how much food our body needed.

As we grew older this inner wisdom became lost in a bewildering host of other inner and outer voices that told us how we *should* eat. We received conflicting messages from our parents, from our peers, from advertising and health classes, from scientific research and diet doctors, and from movies and mirrors. These messages created a confusion of desires, rules, and inner criticism that have rendered us unable to just eat, and to eat just enough.

If we are to return to a healthy and balanced relationship with food, it is essential that we learn to turn our awareness inward and to hear again what our body is always telling us about its needs and its satisfactions. To learn to listen to cellular hunger is a primary skill of mindful eating.

In the autumn you may become aware of "cold hunger," a seasonal aspect of cellular hunger. As the temperature drops the body begins to call for more food. Until recent times, when humans began living in well-heated houses, listening and responding to this demand was essential to our survival. We needed to add a layer of insulating fat to keep our inner organs warm. We needed more calories for the work of keeping the inner furnace going. In particular, women who were pregnant or nursing needed extra calories and extra fat stores in case of food shortage.

When we are sick, we are able to "hear" the requests from our cells. As we recover from the stomach flu, our cells are not interested in a banana split with double fudge sauce or a greasy hamburger. They might tell us, "Just some clear soup and soda crackers." When we have a bad cold, they might declare, "I need orange juice."

deeper lessons

The body has its own wisdom and can tell us a lot about what it requires—if we are able to listen. Unfortunately, as we get older we become deaf to what our bodies are telling us we need. Our mouth demands the sweet taste of candy, our heart asks for mashed potatoes with gravy just like we had at Thanksgiving, our mind says, "Don't you dare go off your diet!" We forget to consult our body. It is always sending us signals, if we know how to stop and pay attention.

The sensation that is most commonly confused with hunger is thirst. If you are hungry at an odd hour, try drinking something. If it's a warm and soothing drink, it might also alleviate heart hunger.

Through mindfulness we can become more sensitive to cellular hunger and learn to separate what the body actually needs from what our mouth and mind are demanding. If we stop and listen carefully and often enough, eventually we might be able to do what some animals do—taste a food and "know" it is what we need. We would eat a banana when our cells asked for more potassium; carrots when we needed beta carotene; eggs or meat when we needed protein or iron; oranges or grapefruit when our cells asked for vitamin C; chocolate when we needed magnesium; and flaxseed, purslane, or fish when our body needed omega-3 fatty acids. We would also know the difference between hunger and thirst.

Tuning in to cellular hunger takes time and practice. It will happen. Be patient. Keep asking your body what it needs.

FINAL WORDS

We can train ourselves to listen to what our body is saying in a very simple way. Take a small pause before eating, turn your attention inward, and ask the body what it needs to do its work.

8

mind hunger

the exercise

Become aware of what the mind is telling you about food and drink. Listen for the mind's comments on what you "should" eat or drink and "should not" eat or drink. Notice whether there are competing voices that say different things about the same food. For example, the mind might be saying, "I'm really thirsty. I'd like a Coke." Another voice says, "Coke is bad for you. Don't you remember, you can dissolve a tooth in Coke! Get juice instead." Another internal voice interrupts to say, "You don't need the calories." Another voice says, "But you do need the caffeine. You're falling asleep at the wheel. Get a Diet Coke." Yet another voice says, "You're addicted to caffeine. You should be able to stay awake without it. Start your caffeine fast right now."

Before you eat, pause and look at your food. Listen inwardly to hear what the mind is saying about the food and drink that is before you.

reminding yourself

Post a picture of a brain or a note saying "What is my mind saying about food?" in various places, including where you usually eat or snack.

discoveries

Mind hunger is based upon thoughts. These thoughts include information, numbers, instructions, and criticism.

"I should eat more protein."

"I deserve an ice cream cone."

"That magazine article said I should drink twelve glasses of water a day."

"Eggs are good for you. They have lots of protein and vitamin A."

"Eggs are bad for you. They have too much cholesterol."

"You ate something that was not on your diet. You are a hopeless failure."

Mind hunger is influenced by what we take in through eyes and ears, the words we read and hear. Thousands of cookbooks provide food for mind hunger. Thousands of diet books provide food for mind hunger.

The voices that make up mind hunger are important to hear but should be taken with a large grain of salt. (But not too large, as salt is currently considered "bad.") "You should start the day with a big breakfast." "You should eat six times a day." "To burn fat, you should skip breakfast so you are fasting for eighteen hours." "Sugar is poison."

The notion that we should eat scientifically and that food is medicine is uniquely American. It leads us to wait anxiously for pronouncements arising from the latest research studies, and to follow the newest fad diet, especially if it is promoted by a telegenic doctor and adopted by a movie star. The food and beverage industry, alert to these trends, develops new products and feeds our anxiety about eating through their advertising.

The journalist Michael Pollan writes in his *New York Times Magazine* article "Our National Eating Disorder":

> We've learned to choose our foods by the numbers (calories, carbs, fats, RDA's, price, whatever), relying more heavily on our reading and computational skills than upon our senses. Indeed, we've lost all confidence in our senses of taste and smell, which can't detect the invisible macro- and micronutrients science has taught us to worry about, and which

food processors have become adept at deceiving anyway. The American supermarket—chilled and stocked with hermetically sealed packages bristling with information—has effectively shut out the Nose and elevated the Eye.

No wonder we have become, in the midst of our astounding abundance, the world's most anxious eaters.

I would suggest that we have actually shut out the nose and elevated the mind. It is the mind that makes us anxious, not the nose or eye. The mind thinks that the body would cooperate and eat perfectly if it could keep us informed about the truth, the scientific nutritional facts. Yet these "facts" are revealed as impermanent, a moving target, changing as new studies are published or when a new medical guru appears. In my childhood butter was "good." In medical school we were taught it was "bad," so doctors recommended switching to margarine. In the last few years we discovered that margarine contains trans fats, so butter is now "good" again. These medical reversals can create a condition of chronic anxiety. When the mind is fretting about "should eat" and "should not eat," our enjoyment of what is actually in our mouth evaporates.

deeper lessons

When we ingest food, the body retains what it needs and excretes the rest. This is not true of our minds.

Everything we put into our minds is retained. If you go to a movie and then to a meditation retreat, you will experience flashes of scenes in the movie for several days. We don't usually detect those lingering traces because our minds are so active, but they are there. They may even surface again several years later in dreams or during meditation.

Meditation is a way of cleaning the storehouse of the mind. As you sit and the mind settles, old memories rise to the surface, like bubbles in a pot on the stove. Some of them will be quite unpleasant, but if you don't react, if you let them arise, exist, and disappear, you will not be adding karmic traces to those memories. If you don't try to either get rid of the memory or cling to it and relive it over and over, its power will diminish. It may arise again, but eventually it will dissolve and disappear. Gradually your mind will become clearer and lighter.

Our minds are nourished and expanded by taking in new information and making new discoveries. If you think about what you read and hear as food for your mind, you may change your habitual patterns of media consumption. Ponder what would be healthier for your mind—"reality" shows or documentaries? Biographies or gossip magazines? A steady diet of news stories about disasters around the world or stories about human kindness, courage, and generosity? Just as the body grows in accord with the food it is fed, so the mind grows in accord with what it takes in. You might undertake a short media fast and see how it affects your peace of mind. (See "A Media Fast," page 85.)

The mind has two functions, thinking and awareness. You can't do both fully at the same time. Mindful eating involves letting go of thoughts and opening all the senses. Here is a motto for life:

Awareness brings intimacy, and intimacy brings a simple happiness—into whatever we are doing.

FINAL WORDS

You can think about food or you can be fully aware of what you are eating. The latter is much more enjoyable and satisfying!

heart hunger

the exercise

When, between meals, you feel the impulse to have a snack or a drink, please look at what emotions you were feeling or what thoughts you were thinking just *before* that impulse arose.

If you have the snack or drink, do those thoughts or emotions change?

reminding yourself

Post a picture of a heart or put a note saying "heart hunger" in your lunch box or in the places you usually eat or snack.

discoveries

Heart hunger is based upon emotions, memories, times of celebration, and feelings of loneliness or connection. I became aware of heart hunger through the comments of participants in our mindful eating workshops. They talked longingly of foods they had eaten for family holidays, foods their mothers had made for them when they were ill, foods eaten with people they loved. It was clear that the particular foods were not as important as the mood or emotion they evoked. Hunger for these foods arose from the desire to be loved and cared for. The memory of those special times infused these foods with warmth and happiness.

How we react emotionally to any food is determined by our past experiences. For example, research shows that when graduate students from China come to the United States to study, cookies are not a comfort food for them. However, after a year of convivial times at parties where cookies are served, cookies have become a comfort food. At our monastery, when we asked people to notice what they were feeling right before they felt the urge to snack, people discovered an array of emotions, including frustration, sadness, irritation, boredom, anxiety, disappointment, anger, confusion, insecurity, and impatience. Notice that these emotions all fall into the category of negative or aversive feelings.

This finding raises some interesting questions. Do we often eat in order to change an uncomfortable state of our mind or heart? Do we eat to soothe ourselves, to get rid of, or at least to cover up, uncomfortable feelings?

Not always, because sometimes we eat because we feel happy or want to celebrate.

Many people in the workshops on mindful eating tell us that they feel a huge hole in their heart. They might relate it to the death of a beloved person or animal. It might be experienced as sadness or as alienation, the feeling of not quite belonging or fitting anywhere. The First Noble Truth of Buddhism is that to live as a human being is to experience suffering. For most of us, it is not the suffering of being caught in war or tortured. It is subtler. As a teenaged girl told me sadly, "I always feel like something is wrong, but I don't know what it is. And I don't know how to fix it." There can be an underlying, pervasive, restless feeling of fundamental unsatisfactoriness. There is a gap between you and the rest of the world. You chat with people, but you don't really connect or feel happy. You eat, but you don't really taste or enjoy.

Many people are aware that they eat in an attempt to fill a hole, not in the stomach but in the heart. Often this habit began in childhood, when we had few tools to cope with the distress in our family. Food was available, an unfailing friend, even if we had to sneak it. Eating is a way we try to take care of ourselves. But we must understand that food put into the stomach will never ease the emptiness or the ache in our heart.

deeper lessons

A woman at a workshop choked up as she told of being in a puzzling transition. She was an excellent cook, and for many years she had taken great pride in feeding her husband and three boys home-cooked meals. Now her sons were grown. The last time they had come home, they said, "Mom, you are always so busy cooking and serving us that you never sit down with us at the table. Come sit down." She couldn't understand why they weren't interested in her food anymore.

I told her, "When they were boys, you fed their stomachs and, at the same time, their hearts, because you cooked with love. Now they are men who can buy whatever they wish to feed the hunger of their stomachs. Now they know that life passes quickly and that time together is precious. They are asking that you sit down and be present with them, talk, tell stories, and laugh with them. They are asking for time with you, time that will nourish the hunger of their hearts."

When you talk with people at any length about comfort foods, you will always uncover a story that is warm with feelings of connection, love, and companionship. All the rich food in the world will not fill our heart's hunger. The heart is nourished by intimacy with ourselves and intimacy with others.

We cannot always depend upon others to fulfill our desire for intimacy, however, because people are always changing. They move away, they fall out of love with us and in love with someone else, they get Alzheimer's and think we are a stranger, and eventually they die.

We need to know how to feed the heart without using food. There are many ways: being in nature, playing with a pet or a child, meditating or saying a centering prayer, doing creative work in any medium—music, wood, dance, clay, fabric, or paints. What is yours? Here's a hint. In the activities that feed your heart, you lose track of time. And when you "come back" into time, you feel refreshed. Please find ways—even small ones—to nourish your heart every day.

We cannot rely on food to fill the empty place in our heart. Ultimately what must nourish our heart is intimacy with this very moment. We often call times of sudden intimacy "peak moments." Some might believe that they happen by accident. In truth, that kind of intimacy is always available. If we stop moving and thinking, let go of past and future, and open all our senses wide, it is right here. We can learn to experience this intimacy with anything that offers itself to us—people or plants, rocks, rice, or raisins. This is what a peak moment brings us to, the sweet and sour and poignant taste of true presence.

When this presence fills us, all hungers vanish. All things, just as they are, are perfect satisfaction.

FINAL WORDS

We will not find full satisfaction in food, no matter how delicious, if we do not nourish the heart on a daily basis. Conversely, when we are mindful with eating, a feeling of intimacy and connection will arise. Then any food can nourish the heart.

10

putting it all together: who's hungry in there?

the exercise

Once you have practiced with each of the Nine Hungers, you can ask this important question: who's hungry in there? When you sit down to eat, pause briefly to do a quick assessment of the Nine Hungers. On a scale of zero to ten, rate each of these: eye, touch, ear, nose, mouth, stomach, cellular, mind, and heart hungers. When you're still new to the practice, you can leave out touch and ear hunger if that's easier.

Once you are aware of the rating for each aspect of hunger, you can make an informed decision about which foods to eat and how much of each food to eat.

reminding yourself

Place a note saying "9 Hungers" or a picture of each body part in your lunch box or near where you usually sit down to eat.

discoveries

If you practice assessing the nine aspects of hunger, you will learn to do this evaluation quite quickly. In fact, someone sitting at the table with you might not even notice. Once you learn to investigate who inside you is hungry, and make it a regular routine to stop and do this exercise before you eat, then you can make a wise and compassionate decision about whether to eat or not. And, if you decide to eat, you can make a better decision about which foods to eat and how much.

If you remember to do this quick assessment again halfway through the meal and especially before taking second helpings, it can be very helpful in adjusting the amount of food you eat to meet your body's *actual* needs.

When people learn to review the Nine Hungers quickly, they are surprised at what they discover. They may feel that they are hungry, but their stomach is saying, "I'm still working on the meal we had an hour ago. Please give me a break!" Or they begin drinking a soda and their mouth says, "No, that's making me feel all sticky and even more thirsty. Please give me plain ice water or hot tea." Or they find that their mouth is clamoring for a taste of something sweet, but their cells are saying, "No, thanks! Remember, sugar gives us a little boost, but then we crash. Our body gets shaky and our mind gets fuzzy. What we need now is some protein to last us through the morning. How about some nuts?"

What do you do then? This is the most interesting aspect of mindful eating. What do you do when you get conflicting information as you assess the nine aspects of hunger?

deeper lessons

Once you are aware of the information from the Nine Hungers, you have choices. Once you have choices, you have stepped into freedom. This is a motto for life:

Awareness brings choice, and choice brings freedom.

When you learn to pop up into awareness—when you can ask, "Who's hungry in there?"—you are no longer a creature chained to old habits. You begin the journey to freedom.

It's like a bus driver with nine unruly passengers. Each passenger is telling you how to drive (faster, slower) and where to go (go to the mall; no, take me home). The bus driver can't react emotionally to all of this input. The driver has to listen, take into account what each passenger is saying, and then make an informed, wise, and compassionate decision about how to drive and where to go. Just so, through mindful eating, you, the driver of the vehicle called your body, will learn to listen to the information from the nine aspects of hunger and make an informed, wise, and compassionate decision about what and where and how much and how fast to eat.

Let's say you have eaten and you are ready to decide about having a second helping. You check in with the nine aspects of hunger. Eyes say, "I love the red color of the strawberries we just ate." The mouth says, "I agree, let's have another strawberry shortcake with lots of whipped cream. I love the contrast of flaky pastry, juicy berries, and smooth, fatty whipped cream." The stomach says, "I'm very full and I have over an hour of work to do to process what you've already given me. Remember how uncomfortable being overfull feels?" The cells say, "We've had plenty of good nutrients and enough fat. No need for more." The mind says, "Are you kidding? Don't be a pig. You've had enough!" The heart says, "I feel soothed by desserts, so let's have more."

Then you, from the spacious place of awareness, take into account the input from these aspects of hunger. You make a decision to have three more strawberries and a small dollop of whipped cream, and to eat slowly and with full attention on what your own wisdom and compassion have chosen. When eating in this way the experience is intimate and satisfying (and does not bring on the hangover of regret and recrimination that an entire shortcake would have created).

Mindful eating helps us step out of automatic pilot and into awareness. Once we are in awareness, the anxiety that has come to flavor our eating dissipates and is replaced by curiosity, discovery, pleasure—and even joy.

FINAL WORDS

When we are aware of all the aspects of hunger, we can make a wise decision about what to eat and how much to eat. When we are not swept away by the demands of the mouth or the whims of the heart, we gain confidence about our ability to eat mindfully and take better care of ourselves.

part two

investigation

Mindful eating is based upon several important changes. One of them involves the inner critic, the voice inside that keeps careful track of our faults and mistakes and angrily berates us about them. Instead of relying on the inner critic to scold or even verbally abuse us when we make food choices it doesn't approve of, we turn to inner investigation and curiosity. In mindful eating, you are simultaneously the scientist, the experimental animal, and the experimental environment. As the experimental animal (you) eats, the curious scientist (you) observes and notes what is occurring in your body, heart, and mind (the experimental environment).

This is one of the most interesting explorations and adventures you can undertake—the exploration of the inner workings of your own unique self. In Zen practice we contemplate the fundamental question (koan), who am I? Or, what is this phenomenon I call my self? How does it work? In mindful eating we make many discoveries that give us clues about some of the answers.

Scientists make new discoveries about food every day. I've been practicing mindful eating for decades, and I'm always making new discoveries. Try it for yourself!

11

trying a new fruit

the exercise

Find a fruit you have never eaten. An Asian food market is a good place to look. Star fruit, lychee, kiwano, rambutan, papaya, custard apple, mangosteen, and dragon fruit are some possibilities. At a Mexican market look for mamey, guanabana, sapote, chico, or pitahaya. Ask to make sure they are ripe.

Sit down with the new fruit and investigate it with all your senses, using the Nine Hungers as a guide. (This is a great way to introduce mindful eating and the nine aspects of hunger to children.) Take it in with your eyes, like a piece of sculpture. For each hunger, ask, "What do I notice? How would I describe this to someone else?" Next, cut it open. What do you see? Smell it. Touch the outer skin and inner fruit. Take a piece in your mouth and roll it around a bit so you can distinguish the flavors. Put full attention in your mouth as you chew and swallow. Does your mouth want more? Now ask your stomach if it wants more. Ask your cells or organs if they like this fruit. Ask your mind if it wants you to try more. Why or why not? Ask your heart if it finds this fruit soothing or comforting.

reminding yourself

Put "new fruit" on your shopping list. Or post on your social media a photo of fruit and your experience with eating it mindfully.

discoveries

If you lived one thousand years ago, you would have no scientific equipment to analyze the nutritional content of a potential food. You would have only the experience of your sense organs and the experience of others. ("Don't eat that fruit. It made Joe sick and die.") If you buy a strange fruit or vegetable in a modern market, you have the assurance that many people have tried it, liked it, and survived, and that there is even a demand for it.

I suggested an unknown *fruit* because humans are born with a liking for sweet foods. Also, you can eat a fruit raw. You could also try this exercise with unknown vegetables such as kohlrabi, chayote squash, oca tubers, tamarillo, or Romanesco, but you will need to find out how to prepare and cook them (something easily done on the internet).

When I try this exercise with children, some are courageous and eager to investigate. "Oh, cool! This is going to be fun!" And some are timid or resistant. "It looks yucky. I'm *not* going to taste it." When they see another child try a bite and enjoy it, however, they may join in. We have those same voices inside our adult heads too. We can all fall into the safe habit of eating the same thing over and over.

We think we have certain innate food preferences, but the only inborn preferences are a liking for sweet and an aversion toward bitter flavors. We are conditioned to like certain foods. This begins with what our mothers ate before we were born. Amniotic fluid takes on the flavor of foods the mother eats, so what mother eats, baby tastes. If mothers eat particular foods or spices, such as garlic, their babies will prefer those foods and flavors after they are born. As the food writer and author Bee Wilson said in a 2016 episode of *Fresh Air*, "Imagine swimming around in that [garlicy amniotic fluid] for nine months. That baby will grow up to love garlic . . . It feels like home, it tastes like home."

The same is true of breast milk. In one study, when mothers drank carrot juice in the last weeks before giving birth or when breastfeeding, their infants later more readily accepted and showed more enjoyment of carrot-flavored cereal than infants who were not exposed to carrot flavor in their amniotic fluid or breast milk. Perhaps forever after, carrots will taste like love.

deeper lessons

Our attitude toward eating a new fruit can reveal something about our attitude toward life. Buddhists divide people into three categories, based upon the "three poisons": greed, anger, and ignorance. These three, if allowed to run unchecked, can poison our experience of life and bring much suffering to us and those around us.

A person who is a "greed" or desire type loves novelty, variety, and new experiences. They might be excited about the opportunity to try an unknown fruit. However, the downside is that they are easily bored and can feel restless and unhappy if the menu of life is not always bringing new "tastes." The positive side of greed is a strong desire to learn.

A person who is an "anger" type is averse to change and novelty. They might be cautious about trying an unknown fruit. They often react to new ideas or suggestions with, "Yes, but . . . " or with a reason why it won't work. The downside is that they make decisions according to what is the least aversive alternative rather than for positive reasons, and can become depressed, with a constricted life. The positive side of aversion is appropriate caution in the face of something new.

A person who is an "ignorance" type reacts to new situations with indifference, apathy, or dissociation, saying, "Whatever . . ." or "I can't be bothered to try." They might choose to remain uninvolved in the exercise of trying a new food. The downside is that they miss out on new experiences and, most important, they can miss out on the experience of being present for their life— the difficulties, lessons, and joys of a unique human life. The positive side of ignorance is "beginner's mind" and the willingness to not know.

Once at the monastery I presented this typology of personality types. One person said, "That is *so* interesting, I'd like to read more about it." The next person said, "I don't agree with that *at all*." I asked someone who was silent what she thought, and she said, "Huh? Oh, I didn't really pay attention to what you were saying." Everyone else laughed.

Each type has its own basic strategy for being safe, successful, and loved in life. All of us have aspects of all three, but can you tell—even from your eating habits— which type sounds like you? Do you crave new tastes and eating experiences? Are you averse to many or new foods? Do you check out while eating and retreat into thoughts about past and future or fantasies? Would you like to change or expand your strategy?

FINAL WORDS

Our attitude toward new foods can reveal our underlying strategies for life. Awareness of our own strategies brings choice, and choice brings freedom, including the choice to be compassionate toward other people who are also boxed in by old strategies.

12

what is your tongue doing now?

the exercise

While eating or drinking, become aware of your tongue. Pause periodically and ask yourself, "What is my tongue sensing or doing right now?" If you have difficulty noticing what your tongue is doing, stop it from moving and then slowly start it up again, almost like a freeze frame, moving it one step at a time. Watch carefully how it works. Or try chewing without moving your tongue, and see what happens. Then bring your tongue back online slowly to investigate how it is involved in chewing.

reminding yourself

Put a picture of a tongue or a note saying "What is my tongue doing?" in the places you usually eat or drink.

discoveries

This is such an interesting exercise. We find that our tongue is a busy little creature! Although it lives right inside our head, ordinarily we ignore it completely—unless we bite or burn it. I sometimes encourage people to make a list of all the jobs of the tongue and see how many they can find. Besides asking how it helps us chew (which is fascinating to watch), you can ask yourself many more questions: How does it get food off a fork and into your mouth? Does it go on top of the fork or underneath? How does it help move liquid from a cup into your mouth? How is it involved in swallowing? How does it decide that it's OK to swallow now? You may need again to slow the process down and ask the tongue, "Are you ready to swallow yet?" If it says "no," then ask, "Why not?" What are its criteria for "ready to swallow"? What does it do after you finish eating?

Even when you are not eating, you can bring attention to the tongue to discover what that little "person" inside your mouth is up to now. What is it doing while you are reading these words? It seldom rests. Over the many years I've done this exercise, I've always discovered new things about the life and loves of my tongue.

After bringing awareness to their tongue, people often express a feeling of gratitude. They realize how difficult life—eating, speaking—would be without a tongue and how cruel the ancient punishment of cutting off tongues actually was.

deeper lessons

Once you become aware of your tongue, you realize that it seldom rests. Between meals it is doing its janitorial duties, checking out your teeth, making sure there are no food particles stuck there or new rough spots. A researcher told me that when we are thinking, our tongue is subtly moving. One way to ease your mind and deepen your meditation is to relax your tongue and let it lie still in your mouth. During meditation I sometimes spread my tongue out so it rests between my back teeth. It helps keep it still and prevents me from unconsciously clenching my jaw. Our tongue has always been with us, has always been taking care of us, since before we were born. (As fetuses, we swallowed amniotic fluid, which helped develop our tongue and digestive tract.) We ignore it most of our lives, but when we bring attention to it, a new world, previously hidden, opens up to us, and gratitude for its untiring service naturally emerges.

Just so, what we call our "True Nature" or "Presence" or "The Great Mystery" (Buddhist terms for the mystery at the heart of all things—you could call it another name, perhaps "God" or the "spirit within") has been dwelling inside of us, closer than our tongue, taking care of us since before we were born. And yet we ignore it most of our lives. When we are suffering—because of our disconnection from it—that very discomfort can catalyze the start of a search for what we feel we have lost.

And when we step on the spiritual path, and begin to experience its unvarying presence in so many aspects of our lives, we realize that—just like our tongue—our True Nature is always functioning, from within us. It also functions through us, to help those who also suffer in the world. This discovery opens a new appreciation for the unfolding mystery of existence and a feeling of deep gratitude for our part in it.

FINAL WORDS

Your tongue works to care for you continually. Just as surely as you were able to see what your tongue is doing, if you keep walking your spiritual path, you will experience the Presence of this Great Mystery at work within your own body, heart, mind, and life.

13

a media fast

the exercise

For one week, do not take in any media. This includes news media, social media, and entertainment. Do not listen to the radio, iPods, or CDs; don't watch TV, films, or video; don't read newspapers, books, or magazines (whether online or in print form); don't surf the internet and don't check Facebook or Twitter.

You don't have to plug your ears if someone tells you about a news event, but do avoid being drawn in to a conversation about the news. If people insist, tell them about your unusual kind of fast. You may, of course, do reading or answer those e-mails that are necessary for work or school.

What to do instead? Discovering alternatives to consuming media is part of this mindfulness practice. Hint: do something with your own hands and your own body.

Live your own life instead of becoming lost in someone else's.

reminding yourself

Cover the TV with a sheet, put a sign on your car radio and computer screen reminding you "no news or entertainment this week." Let magazines accumulate and consider putting newspapers straight into recycling. You could do this if you went on vacation—why not now?

discoveries

I invented this task for a student who suffered from a very common problem, chronic low-level anxiety. At the end of a six-day silent retreat he shared his happiness over his calm state of mind. An hour later at lunch, however, I heard him fuming, as usual, about the terrible state the world was in. An admitted news junkie who grew up in New York City, he undertook a media fast with great reluctance. He discovered that his state of mind was good upon arising and while doing his early morning meditation. But as soon as the meditation ended, his habit was to grab a cup of coffee and turn on the morning news, "so I can see how the bastards have messed up now." During the media fast, he was surprised to find that if he wasn't up on the latest news, it didn't really matter, at home or at work. He was, however, experiencing a much calmer state of mind, and his patient wife was extremely grateful.

What we see on TV influences our mind and heart. It can set the mood for our day or our perception of what is normal. Research shows that children exposed to violence on TV are more likely to act violently soon after. Some young adults believe that if they are not living a life that is as exciting as a soap opera or a reality show—filled with the drama of hot romance, angry breakups, mistaken identities, and kidnappings—then their life is somehow flawed.

One challenge during a media fast is finding an activity to substitute for the time usually spent with the media. You can meditate, take a walk, play a game with your family, cook something from scratch, weed the garden, take photos, do artwork, learn a new language, play a musical instrument, or just sit on the porch and relax.

You might discover that not knowing the latest news makes you feel powerless, fearful, or stupid. People ask me, "What if something important happens, like a fire or a terrorist bombing?" I say, "Don't worry, if it's that important someone will tell you about it."

deeper lessons

I was in a silent seven-day retreat when someone came in to the meditation hall and quietly told us about the

9/11 tragedy. A few people left the hall briefly to call and check on relatives in New York City. We continued to sit in the truth of not being able to affect the outcome, and we chanted and prayed for everyone impacted by the disaster. Afterward we heard about the repetitive trauma experienced by people who had watched the disaster play out on TV, over and over, for days. There is little we can do about most tragedies in the world. But we can stay calm and pray.

Here is my algebra of suffering. If there is N amount of suffering in the world, and we suffer because of hearing about it, now there is N+1 amount of suffering in the world. If a paramedic arrived at the scene of a car crash and went into hysterics over how terrible it was, it would be no help. It would only add to the distress of the event. Is our goal to reduce or increase suffering?

For the first two hundred thousand years of human history, we were exposed to the news (and the pain) of only those immediately around us in our tribes and villages. We saw birth, sickness, death, and wars, but on a limited scale. Just in the last forty years or so has the news media—first the nightly news, now 24/7 cable news—poured the suffering of the entire world into our ears and eyes, every day, day after day. Murder, torture, genocide, deadly epidemics, wars, natural disasters, starvation—our hearts and minds were not designed to take in this much anguish. The world is flawed, millions of innocent people suffer, and we are unable to do much to change it. This suffering accumulates in our minds and hearts and makes us suffer in turn. When the mind and heart become too full of pictures of violence, destruction, and pain, we must take time to empty ourselves.

A media fast is one way to do this. A silent retreat is even better.

If we can decrease our intake of these toxic images, we can more easily establish a compassionate heart and a mind that is serene and clear. This is the best foundation we can have to move out into the world of woe, meet whatever comes toward us, and be of benefit.

FINAL WORDS

Your mind is shaped by the information you feed it. Choose its food wisely. A steady diet of negative news makes the mind and heart sick. Give them the good nourishment of silence, time alone in nature, beauty, and loving friendship.

14

it's ok to be empty

the exercise

Sit quietly for a few minutes and bring awareness to your body. Are there places in the body that feel empty? Are the sensations of emptiness pleasant, neutral, or unpleasant? Are there places in the body that feel full? Are the sensations of fullness pleasant, neutral, or unpleasant? Do any impulses arise to change the sensations of emptiness or fullness in the body?

Repeat this investigation several times during the day and before going to bed.

reminding yourself

Post notes saying "Empty?" in several places in your home and at work.

discoveries

Do you think there is something wrong if you feel hungry? Do you keep emergency stashes of food in your purse or briefcase, your car, or your office drawer, just in case your stomach starts to growl? I do. When I'm on the go and find myself hungry, I know that somewhere, deep in the recesses of my purse, there are three-year-old mints, covered with fuzz, and a stale energy bar—just in case my plane crashes and I'm washed up on an uninhabited sandy island or if I'm abducted by terrorists who are impolite enough to forget to feed me at my regular mealtimes.

In modern Western culture we seem to be very uncomfortable with the collection of sensations that we call "hunger" or "thirst." We keep a drink always at hand. We snack all day long. We say, "Actually, I'm not very hungry," and proceed to eat an entire meal, in order to make sure that we won't feel hungry later. When we become aware of the intense energy behind this constant filling behavior, we have to ask a question: am I willing to be empty? Most people answer "no." They like the feeling of fullness in their abdomen. It is comforting. As they investigate mindful eating, they may discover that when they feel empty, fear arises. They may find that they are eating and drinking all day long in order to avoid this feeling. They are imprisoned by the desire for the mouth and stomach to feel full.

Other people, however, answer, "Yes, I like feeling empty." For them the feeling of emptiness in their abdomen is pleasant. The feeling of fullness is unpleasant. After eating they may vomit, purge, or take enemas in order to empty the body and get rid of the feeling of fullness. They are imprisoned by aversion to the feeling of being full.

Other people answer, "I don't know." They are unaware of whether their stomach or body is signaling hunger. They eat by the clock, or they eat when and how much the herd eats. Distracted by media, they are unaware of what they are eating. They are imprisoned by ignorance.

When we eat and drink all the time, our stomach and all our other digestive organs never get a rest. When we never let ourselves become truly hungry, our enjoyment of food decreases. Isn't it ironic? We think that by eating more we are enjoying eating more, but this is not true. It is when we allow ourselves to become truly hungry, to take time to eat slowly and with attention, to stop when we are comfortably full (or a little less) that we find the most enjoyment in eating.

deeper lessons

The First Noble Truth of Buddhism is the universality of suffering. If you are a human being, you will encounter suffering in your life. Many people in industrialized countries hear this and think, "The truth of suffering doesn't apply to me. I'm not in a war zone, I'm not being tortured or starving." The suffering that the Buddha talked about, however, is an experience that is often much subtler than outright pain. It is a sense of dissatisfaction, a persistent feeling that things are not as they should be. Sometimes it's the feeling that your life is empty. It is an unpleasant feeling, one that impels us to move, to do something, to distract ourselves, to eat something, to drink something, to buy something, or to binge to make the feeling of dis-ease go away.

Moving away and creating distractions are not long-term solutions to this feeling that something is not right. It is a feeling based in truth. It must be attended to. Eating, drinking, using drugs or alcohol, risking danger, courting a new lover—these are all over-the-counter remedies for temporary relief of this fundamental dis-ease, the intuition that things are not as they could or even should be. The true source of this dissatisfaction is spiritual, and thus the only true cure for it is also spiritual.

Are you willing to be empty? Now we need to look at the question from the spiritual point of view. First of all, we *are* empty, whether we like it or not. Every atom in our body is composed of emptiness (more than 99 percent) inhabited by tiny bits of whizzing energy (less than 1 percent).

In addition to our very real physical emptiness, we are empty in another way. We are empty of independent existence. We could not exist without all other beings also existing. Sometimes we become overwhelmed by the multitude of "others" and might wish that everything else in the world would disappear, but if that happened, we too would disappear. Fundamentally we are made up of our interactions with all other beings. We are each like a soap bubble in the middle of a huge mass of soap bubbles. We are made up of nothing but emptiness and our intersections and interactions with all the other beings. And so are they.

To be willing to be empty is to align with a fundamental truth of our being.

Similarly, when we think all the time, our minds never get a rest. Here too emptying is as important as filling. Life-changing insights arise out of a mind that is calm and aware. This emptying is the essence of centering prayer or meditation. God can't call in on a busy line.

FINAL WORDS

Emptying is as important as filling. For the body and the mind.

part three

loving-kindness

Did you ever notice that you're not perfect? Thank goodness we're not. Would you like to be married to a perfect person? No, shudder at the thought. We could never measure up. It's the little imperfections that make us unique, cute, charming, interesting, and loveable.

Except to ourselves. The inner critic is the name we give to the voice inside of us that is very worried, or even frantic, about our ability to survive, be loved, and become successful. The inner critic has only one tool, criticism. Our inner critic hates that we are not perfect. It is constantly berating us, hoping that its angry words will magically change us into perfect . . . what? Robots programmed into perfection? The inner critic uses anger to try to change us, but anger is not a good way to bring about change. It only causes us to react with anger or fear and despair.

In mindfulness we replace the inner critic with investigation and curiosity. With mindful eating we are the inquisitive scientist investigating the research animal, which is also us. For researchers the mistakes, the imperfections, the surprises, and the failures are the most intriguing. If we stay with these imperfect qualities and look deeper, we can often uncover something very interesting—how our body and our personality work. We can detect our hidden beliefs and habit patterns, see where our suffering comes from, and learn how to dissolve it.

Loving-kindness is the specific antidote to anger and fear. We can direct it toward ourselves, toward our body. This is not a selfish thing to do (as the inner critic might complain). Rather, it is a necessary thing to do if we want to help others. We can direct it toward others who are suffering just as we are. We can even direct it toward the neurotic, fearful inner critic. Loving-kindness is a vital form of nourishment that all living beings require to thrive.

15

treat yourself as a guest

the exercise

Make a mindful meal once a day, treating yourself as if you were a guest. You could get out your best plates and silverware, a place mat or tablecloth, even a small vase of flowers and a candle. Arrange food appealingly, as if for a guest. As you eat, let your eyes "feed" on not only the food but also the other aspects of your table. Eat at least the first few bites mindfully, as if savoring the food your kind host has provided.

Even when you have a snack, you can take time to make it attractive. Arrange apple slices in a fan or tangerine segments in a star shape on a napkin or plate, and add a leaf or flower.

reminding yourself

Before you eat, gather the accessories you might use for a meal with a guest—a place mat on a tray, a vase of flowers, attractive bowls and plates. If those accessories are out of cupboards and visible, it will help remind you to use them. You can also post a note saying "I'm the guest" in places where you commonly eat.

discoveries

If she caught us eating standing up, my mother-in-law would say, "This is not a bus station. Please sit down." I realized that even if I am in a hurry, I still have time to sit down to eat, to use nice bowls and plates, and perhaps to set out a few flowers and a place mat. If I catch myself eating while standing at the sink, I at least sit down. Sitting makes me slow down and focus on eating.

My mother and my mother-in-law treated meals, especially supper, as an important, almost sacred time. They always "set a nice table." Since we were all bookworms, my mother forbade us to read at the table, or even to hold a book open under the table where we could sneak a quick peek. Certainly she would have banned cell phones during meals. We talked about the events of our day. Sometimes my mother recited a poem and we discussed what it meant. Sometimes she asked us each to memorize a poem to share at the table.

People attending mindful eating workshops often describe very different experiences around meals. In some families everyone got what they wanted from the fridge and ate alone in their rooms with their TV or computer for company. In others, meals were strained, tense, or even a time for verbal abuse. No wonder it might be difficult as an adult to sit down and take time to eat without distractions. When food has been flavored with anxiety and punishment for years, it takes a while to change that conditioning and be able to pair food with relaxation and pleasure.

There is research showing that a family meal time can have many benefits for growing children. Regular family meals are linked to good self-esteem, resilience, and better grades in children and teens. They also result in lower rates of depression, eating disorders, and substance abuse.

No matter the reason, if you missed the warmth of family meals, if you were not treated as a welcome guest at the table, you can provide this gift to yourself now.

deeper lessons

We have all sorts of excuses for not taking a bit more time to treat ourselves as a guest. But it comes down to this: Do we feel that we deserve to be treated well, as well as a friend or a guest? Do we feel that it would be somehow selfish to take that extra care?

We feed our heart when we take care in preparing food for ourselves, treating ourselves as well as we would a guest. It only takes a few minutes to arrange food nicely on a plate rather than eating out of a cardboard take-home carton, or to sit down at a table you have set with a colorful place mat and candle rather than eating standing up at the refrigerator or the kitchen counter.

Treating ourselves as guests reminds us to stop and appreciate this very moment in our life. We can't rely on other people to provide the support and care we long for. When we become our own best friend, when we enjoy our own company, we are never lonely. When you treat yourself as a guest, when you invite awareness and curiosity to join you, even simple food like oatmeal and milk or a bowl of instant noodles can become much more enjoyable.

Our deepest human longing is for connection. When we take a few extra minutes to treat ourselves kindly, to be present with our food, we are nourishing our heart as well as our body. That is the key to satisfaction. All the rich food in the world will not fill our heart's hunger. The heart is nourished by intimacy with ourselves, and with others.

FINAL WORDS

Become a generous host—treat yourself as an honored guest at the table.

16

loving-kindness for the body

the exercise

This is an exercise to do during a brief meditation. Sit comfortably, close your eyes, and bring awareness to different parts of your body, one part at a time. For example, you could bring awareness to each of the organs involved in the Nine Hungers—your eyes, skin, ears, nose, mouth, stomach, cells, mind (or brain), and heart. Rest your awareness in the sensations arising from that body part (touch, pressure, temperature, sounds, etc.). Before you move on to another body part, you silently direct a wish to it by saying several times, "May you be free from difficulty. May you be at ease. May you be healthy."

reminding yourself

Put a picture of a body with a heart on it in the places where you meditate and on your bed pillow. Even better, print out a photo of yourself and draw a heart on it, and put it in the same places.

discoveries

Loving-kindness is a feeling of basic friendliness. Do you feel basically friendly toward your body? To all its parts? Without knowing it, we can build up resentments toward our body. There are aspects of our body we don't like, such as small eyes, teeth that aren't perfect, ears that stick out, straight or balding hair—it's endless! This is especially true if a body part is having difficulty or not functioning perfectly. Instead of feeling compassion toward our aching head, our nearsighted eyes, our overfull stomach, our bum knee, our strained back, or our stubbed toe, we try to ignore it or feel unconsciously angry toward it.

I once heard a mentor do a body review with a woman, asking her inner critic what was wrong with various body parts, beginning with her hair and moving down. For each body part the inner critic had scathing comments. Her hair? "Her hair is a mess. It's the wrong color, but I don't want her to dye it. Then it would be fake. I want it to be naturally silky and shiny." Her eyes? "Close set and beady. Nothing to be done about it. She looks like a weasel!" Her lips? "Too thin. They should be full and luscious." And so on; for every body part, a criticism. He finally asked her, "Is there one body part that's OK? How about her left little fingernail?" "Well," the inner critic responded grudgingly, "it's a bit too small, but I guess it's OK."

Nothing thrives under a bombardment of negativity, not plants, animals, or children. The same is true of our bodies. All the parts are doing the best they can to support us. Our bodies were designed to last thirty-five to forty years, which was the human life span for most of our two hundred thousand years of evolution. If we are over the age of fifty, and we are still chugging along, we are doing very well!

We worry about those we love, but worry has a negative impact and is not received as the underlying emotion of love. Return to the authentic emotion—affection and care—and channel that. You can send the loving-kindness prayers to anyone or anything you are worried about. "May my son be at ease and happy." "May all injured animals be healed." "May anyone with a headache like mine tonight find relief from their pain."

deeper lessons

Our minds are magnetically attracted toward the negative. Just look at the news. At least 90 percent of it is negative—wars, murders, child abuse, toxins, outbreaks of life-threatening diseases, climate destruction, athletic doping, extinction of another species, and political corruption. Here and there you find a human-interest story about a lost puppy who traveled two hundred miles to find its way home. The *New York Times* has a feature on Fridays called "The Week in Good News" to help counterbalance the daily barrage of anxiety-producing news and "send you into the weekend with a smile, or at least a lighter heart."

Our mind wants to keep us safe, so it fixates on potential dangers. It doesn't particularly care about good news because good things can't hurt or kill us. Unfortunately, the mind can also take the same attitude toward our bodies. It ignores what is working well and focuses on what it does not like, such as what might be unattractive, imperfect, or anything it interprets as signs of impending illness or death.

A steady stream of negative thoughts creates an unhappy world to live in. And when the burden of critical thoughts about ourselves becomes intolerable, we tend to let it overflow as criticism of others. This is guaranteed to make our world an even more unpleasant place to live in.

There is medicine for this affliction. It consists of awareness and change. First, we have to become aware of when the mind is headed down the fast-flowing stream of negative thinking, a stream that is headed for a toxic pond of anger and resentment. Then we need to pick up the mind and place it in a new stream, one that is positive and will flow toward a destination that is peaceful and at ease. One of the most effective ways to change the course of the mind-stream is to do loving-kindness practice. It is the specific medicine prescribed by the Buddha for the afflictions of anger, fear, and dread.

FINAL WORDS

When you discover that your mind is sinking toward unhappiness with yourself or with others, that is exactly the right time to do loving-kindness practice.

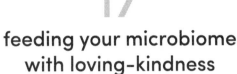

feeding your microbiome with loving-kindness

the exercise

As you take your first bites of food, send them down to the many tiny beings in your gut with kindness, like a parent lovingly feeding their hungry children (lots of them!). You can compose a prayer for them, such as, "May this food give you good health so that the body that is your dwelling place can also be healthy." Every few bites, or as you start eating seconds, you can repeat this silent dedication.

reminding yourself

Place a picture or drawing of the microbiome or a note saying "L-K for my microbiome" in your lunch box or where you usually eat.

discoveries

We usually think of our body as a collection of separate organs, including brain, heart, stomach, and liver. We are beginning to realize that we are less like a group of organs and more like a complex universe, a universe that hosts billions of other microscopic beings that interact with all our own cells. These microscopic beings are vital to our health. What we think of as a single being, "myself," actually contains ten times more cells belonging to other beings than human cells. Most of these other beings reside in our gut, but they also live all over our body, in our scalp, noses, eyes, armpits, and belly buttons. They are called the "human microbiome." We have coevolved with them over eons and could not exist without them.

Our organs are not isolated. Just as our brain receives information from, and transmits information to, the entirety of our body, so our gut bacteria seem to be communicating continually with the rest of our body, including our brain and immune system, with messages flowing in both directions. They may even influence what foods we crave. If we eat junk food and thus cultivate gut bacteria that thrive on junk food, might they entice us to eat more junk food?

Researchers are finding associations between an altered gut microbiome and such diverse disorders as diabetes, malnutrition, autism, asthma, eczema, heart disease, irritable bowel syndrome, and a variety of disorders linked to inflammation including cardiovascular disease, inflammatory bowel disease, multiple sclerosis, and some cancers. People who are obese have a different microbiome (fewer numbers and species of bacteria) in their gut than people who are at a healthy weight.

The multitude of beings living in our gut may also play a role in our mental and emotional states. They manufacture some vitamins and neurotransmitters such as serotonin, a natural antidepressant. Ninety percent of the serotonin in our body is found in our gastrointestinal system.

deeper lessons

We are aware that our genes are responsible for much of who we think we are—our height, the color of our skin, hair, and eyes, our body build, and whether we find the taste of cilantro pleasant or disgusting. However, the genetic material inside us is only 1 percent human; the rest belongs to the microbes living on and within our body. This is biological proof of what the Zen teacher Thich Nhat Hahn calls the fact of our "interbeing," that we are literally made up largely of elements we would call "not me."

It adds poignancy to the Zen question, who am I? As we discover more about what these tiny internal beings do, it also makes us wonder, who is in charge of me?

Who is in charge of my health? Who is in charge of my moods? Certainly, it behooves us to take good care of these interbeings inside us.

One way is to eat foods that contain beneficial bacteria. They are commonly called "probiotics" and are found in certain cultured or fermented foods including unpasteurized yogurt, water or milk kefir, kombucha, miso, tempeh, sourdough, and kimchi or true sauerkraut (not cabbage pickled in vinegar).

We should be aware of which foods beneficial microbes thrive on. Their well-being ensures the thriving of their host organisms, meaning you and me. Big surprise! They flourish on whole foods containing fiber—that is, vegetables, whole grains, legumes (lentils, peas, and beans), nuts, and fruits. When we eat well, they eat well, and then we feel well.

FINAL WORDS

Be a loving parent to the many beings inside you. Nourish them well so that they will support the health of your body, heart, and mind.

part four

slowing down

Slowing down is one of the most potent mindful eating practices we can engage in. Americans tend to eat very quickly. Many people have told me that their attitude toward meals is to just get it over with as soon as possible. The American habit of eating fast is not new. Foreigners visiting early American taverns recorded their astonishment at how quickly food was eaten. The technique was dubbed "the three Gs" for "gobble, gulp, and go." The Tennessee historian Dallas Bogan records in "Foods of the Early Tavern and Household" on the *History of Campbell Country, Tennessee* website that a European visiting the colonies was puzzled by the "haste, hustle and starving attitude the inn frequenter displayed. Everyone stuffed himself at uncanny speeds." Our propensity to eat and run has not diminished over the intervening two centuries. Research shows that North Americans spend only eleven minutes eating lunch at a fast-food restaurant and eighteen minutes at a cafeteria in their workplace.

In North America we often eat standing up or while walking or driving, just cramming the food down on our way to do something else. It's as if we want to get eating over with quickly. You can buy a giant bib to wear as you drive so that your work clothes don't get stained by the food you spill as you lurch down the road.

In many Asian and European countries this is considered a shocking way to eat, bordering on barbaric. In Japan it is considered very rude to eat while walking. Even fast food is to be eaten respectfully, sitting down. An ice cream cone is the only exception, because it will melt. When I began teaching mindful eating in Europe, I was surprised to see outdoor cafés full of people at seven and eight o'clock at night, even in cold weather. They were eating, talking, and drinking quite leisurely. A meal is a ceremony, a time to enjoy not just the food but the anticipation of the food, and the good company. To give the food and drink proper attention is to repay the effort of the people who are serving you. You repay them more with your appreciation than with your money.

Research shows that slowing down can be a potent practice. Many studies from around the world on people of all ages confirm that simply slowing down the speed of eating reduces the risk of weight gain (including regaining weight after bariatric surgery), obesity, high blood pressure, high blood sugar, abnormal blood lipids, and metabolic syndrome.

When we introduce the practice of chewing thoroughly, workshop participants often find it a novel experience. One woman exclaimed, "I realized that I barely chew at all! All my life the food has gone in my mouth and down my throat, almost unchanged." How many chews it takes to process your food well depends upon whether you are eating broth (none) or nuts (lots). Experiment with this yourself—try one meal a day where you chew each bite well.

There's an intelligence in eating slowly. Some of our satisfaction in eating comes from chewing. Chewing food well not only gives the mouth more exercise and more satisfaction from experiencing changing textures and flavors; it also helps break down food into smaller particles so we get more nutrients from what we eat. There are enzymes in saliva that break down food, allowing the mouth to begin absorbing nutrients even before we have swallowed, but this enzyme activity will only happen if we actually chew our food and let it stay in the mouth for more than a few seconds.

When food exits the stomach and enters the small intestine, appestat hormones signal the brain and body, "We've had enough. We're satisfied. Time to slow down or stop eating." It takes about twenty minutes for this important biological feedback loop to be completed. If we eat slowly we allow food time to reach the small intestine and trigger the "OK, I'm full" signal before we've eaten too much. If we eat too quickly we've already packed in too much food before the satiation signal can arrive. Then we don't stop eating until we are physically uncomfortable, which is after we've consumed more calories than our body needs.

Don't worry that undertaking mindful eating will condemn you to a life of always eating *very slowly.* It is more difficult to be mindful while eating quickly. But slow down when you can. One woman told me that she picked slowing down as the one mindful eating practice she could do. After slowing her eating down, she lost thirty-five unwanted pounds and also improved her relationship with her partner, a poky eater.

eating with the
non-dominant hand

the exercise

For one week try eating at least part of each meal with your non-dominant hand. You can expand this to include all drinks and more meals each day. If you're up for a big challenge, try using the non-dominant hand to eat with chopsticks.

reminding yourself

Put a picture of a hand with an X through it in your lunch box or near where you usually eat. Or put a Band-Aid on your dominant hand or a rubber band around your wrist to remind you to switch to using your non-dominant hand. You could also place a sign where you eat that says "left hand" (if you are right-handed). Or use an unusual color of nail polish on your non-dominant hand to signal "use me!"

discoveries

This experiment always evokes laughter. We discover that the non-dominant hand is quite clumsy.

This exercise takes us back to what Zen teachers call "beginner's mind." Our dominant hand might be forty years old, but the non-dominant hand feels much younger, perhaps about two or three years old. We have to learn all over again how to hold a fork and how to get it into our mouths without stabbing ourselves. We might begin to eat with the non-dominant hand, and then, when our attention wanders, our dominant hand will reach out and take the fork away. It's just like a bossy older sister who says, "Hey, you little klutz, let me do it for you!"

You can have more fun if you use your non-dominant hand for other everyday tasks such as brushing your teeth or hair, opening doors, writing, or cutting with scissors. You can also try switching the usual roles that each hand plays when they work together. Have the non-dominant hand wield the hammer and do the pounding while the dominant hand holds a nail, or reverse the hands while stirring a pot of food or washing dishes. I've discovered that my right hand is skilled in fine motor movements, but my left hand is the less intelligent "strong woman" who can better hold a baby on my hip or steady the cheese grater while the right hand grates the cheese.

Struggling to use the non-dominant hand can awaken our compassion for anyone who is clumsy or unskilled, such as a person who has had disabilities, injuries, or a stroke. We see briefly how we take for granted scores of simple movements that many people cannot make.

Researchers speculate that one reason that obesity is less common in countries like Japan is that when you eat with chopsticks, you must take small bites. Using chopsticks with the non-dominant hand is a humbling experience. If you want to eat a meal in under an hour and not end up spilling food all over, you have to be very attentive.

deeper lessons

Using the non-dominant hand reveals our impatience. Isn't it interesting that we become impatient with eating, one of the most pleasurable activities we humans engage in? Why are we anxious to get it over with quickly? It's self-defeating!

If each person has one major lesson for each lifetime, mine would be impatience. I've investigated impatience by asking, impatient to get to what? I'm impatient to finish breakfast so I can do what? E-mails. I'm impatient to finish e-mails so I can get to . . . working on this book . . . finishing a ceramic statue . . . eating lunch . . . lying down for a nap. . . . If I continue to carry this forward I discover that I'm impatient to eventually get to what . . . my death?! That realization jolts me back into a more vivid experience and enjoyment of this moment of life, a life I am not at all impatient to leave.

If you step back and simply observe how your two hands work together as a team in routine tasks such as eating or washing dishes, you will see that they work together beautifully, quietly and continually caring for you. If everyone in the world worked together in this way, aiding and supporting one another as they cared for the life of this earth, the world would be an entirely different place.

Using the non-dominant hand can help us become more flexible and discover that we are never too old to learn new tricks. If we practice frequently, over time we can watch our skill develop. I have been practicing using my left hand for several years, and I now forget which hand is the "right" hand to use. This could have practical benefits. If I lose the use of my dominant hand, as a number of my relatives did after strokes, I won't be "left" helpless. When we develop a new skill, we realize that there are many other abilities lying dormant within us.

FINAL WORDS

Simply using your non-dominant hand can invoke beginner's mind and open a world of interesting discoveries.

19

one bite at a time, or put down that utensil!

the exercise

This is a mindfulness practice to do whenever you are eating. After you take a bite, put the fork or spoon back down in the bowl or on the plate. Place your awareness in your mouth until that one bite has been enjoyed and swallowed. Only then do you pick up the utensil and take another bite. If you are eating with your hands, put the sandwich or apple or cookie down between bites.

reminding yourself

Post notes saying "one bite at a time" wherever you eat, or an icon of a spoon or fork with the words "Put it down!"

discoveries

This is one of the most challenging of all the mindful eating practices we do at our monastery. In attempting this exercise, most people discover that they have the habit of "layering" bites of food. That is, they put one bite in the mouth, divert their attention away from the mouth as they shovel food onto the fork or spoon for the next bite, then put a second bite in the mouth before the first one is swallowed. Often the hand is hovering in the air, with another bite halfway to the mouth, as the preceding bite is chewed. They discover that as soon as the mind wanders, the hand assumes control again, putting new bites of food in along with partially processed bites. It is amazing how hard this simple task can be. It takes time, patience, persistence, and a sense of humor to change long-term habits.

Manufacturers of foodlike substances are well aware that we like the hit of intense flavor and texture sensations that occur as soon as we take the first bite of food. They are also aware that as soon as those sensations begin to fade, we will take another bite. And another. The more quickly the sensations disappear, the more of their product we will mindlessly consume. You can try this for yourself. Pick something like cheese puffs or a variety of potato chips that are coated with flavor dust. Put one in your mouth and let it sit there. You can roll it around with your tongue, but don't chew it. What happens to the initial crispy texture and bright flavor? How long does it take for it to become uninteresting or even repulsive? What is your impulse when that happens?

A nurse told me about a woman who was learning to chew her food well, one bite at a time, a necessity following her bariatric surgery. The woman was surprised at what a difference it made, how it enriched and expanded her experience of eating, and said, "If I'd learned this earlier, I wouldn't have needed the surgery!"

Putting down your utensil between bites used to be part of good manners. It counteracts the tendency to wolf down our food. One person exclaimed after trying this task, "I just realized that I never chew my food! I swallow it almost whole, in my haste to get the next bite in." He had to ask himself, "Why am I in such a rush to get through a meal, when I enjoy eating so much?"

deeper lessons

This is another exercise in which we become aware of impatience. Eating quickly, layering one bite on top of another, is a specific example of impatience. Doing this practice may lead you to watch impatience arise in other aspects and occasions in your life. Do you get impatient when you have to wait? We have to ask ourselves, "Why am I in such a rush to get through life, when I want to enjoy it so much?"

Experiencing one bite or one swallow at a time is a way of experiencing one moment at a time. Since we eat or drink at least three times a day, this mindfulness practice gives us several built-in opportunities to bring mindfulness into each day. Eating is naturally pleasurable, but when we eat quickly and without mindfulness, we don't enjoy it. Research shows that people eat their favorite foods more quickly. How self-defeating! Binge eaters also report that they keep on eating in a vain effort to re-create the pleasure of the first bite. Because the taste receptors tire quickly, this will never work. If we want the flavors in each bite to be clear, we need to pause a bit to refresh our taste buds.

When the mind is absent, thinking about the past or future, we are only half tasting our food. When our awareness rests in the mouth, when we are fully present as we eat, when we slow our eating, pausing between bites, then each bite can be like the first—rich and full of interesting sensations.

FINAL WORDS

Pursuing pleasure without mindfulness is like being caught on a treadmill. You eat more but enjoy it less. Mindfulness allows pleasure to bloom in thousands of small moments in your life.

20
saying grace

the exercise

For one week, pause to say grace before you begin eating.
It can be as simple as stopping for a moment to look at
your food and to say silently, "Thank you for this food."
If you are with your family, you can hold hands in silence
for fifteen or twenty seconds while each person silently
thanks the people and other beings who brought the food
to the table. Or it can be a memorized religious prayer.
If you already say grace, try a new one.

reminding yourself

Post notes saying "grace" in your lunch box or in the places
where you usually eat. When appropriate, you can ask
others to join you in a moment of silence to appreciate
the food before digging in.

discoveries

In Japan everyone bows before eating and says, *Itada-kimasu* (I receive this gratefully), and after finishing, *Go-chisosama deshita* (it was delicious). This training begins in childhood. Many people in the West were taught to say grace when they were young. With decreasing participation in formal religion, this seems to be much less common. Research shows that any ritual that helps us pause before eating will help enhance our perception of the food's flavor, increase the time we spend savoring it, and even increase how we value the food—how much we'd be willing to pay for it. The ritual can be as simple as breaking a small candy bar in half and unwrapping and eating each half by itself. Small ceremonies like this bring our awareness to what we are eating rather than what we are thinking, switching us out of automatic pilot and into our actual experience, unclouded by thoughts and fantasies.

Even what seems like nonsense activity works if it helps us pause before eating. In one study people who waited to eat carrots (a four-calorie snack) after knocking on the table twice, picking up the bag of carrots, and then knocking again enjoyed them more than those who did random gestures or had no delay before eating. The effect works only for the person who does the ritual, not for someone who just watches it. The researchers concluded that rituals enhance flavor and enjoyment because they focus people's interest on the food to come. They call this "focus involvement." We call it "deliberately bringing mindful attention to eating."

Research studies also show that cultivating the habit of expressing gratitude during the day increases overall happiness. Why would we resist taking a few moments each time we eat to give thanks if it brought us more happiness and helped us eat more mindfully?

One reason, some say, is that it's embarrassing to bow your head and sit quietly when you are in a restaurant or with people who don't say grace. It can create an awkward silence. I've found, however, that many people in restaurants seem to appreciate seeing someone say grace. Without being terribly obvious, it's easy to look at the plate the waiter has just put in front of me, take the food in with my eyes, and silently say thanks. Sometimes people even ask me to bless the food. If you are at a buffet you can say grace silently as you wait in line.

deeper lessons

It is so easy to move through a fast-paced life without pausing to consider how blessed we are. Those blessings become obvious to us when we do stop, ask, and investigate, "What is being given to me right now?" As we open our senses we become aware of the gift of air, of the oxygen supplied by the plants around us. We become aware of the unfailing support of the earth beneath us—whose presence we take for granted every time we take a step or sit or lie down. Wind, rain, shelter, clothing, electricity, clean water to drink—so many gifts.

At our monastery meals, each person makes a food offering—placing a bit of food on a small plate, saying silently, "May all be equally nourished." This shows our willingness to share what we have with those who are hungry. It is our prayer that everyone in the world will be as well-nourished as we are. We practice expanding our awareness as we pray, beginning with the food, then opening to the people who brought it to us, and finally to everyone in the world, especially those who are hungry.

If you would like to make saying grace a regular practice, here are some samples.

This food is a gift of the whole universe, and the lives of many living beings. May we live so that we are worthy to receive it.

I am grateful for this food, for the earth, the sun, the rain, and all the beings who brought it to me. May I use the blessings of my life to benefit others.

I give thanks for this food. May it bring my mind to greater clarity, my heart to greater love, and my body to greater service.

May those who brought this food to me, and everyone
I meet today, find peace, justice, and happiness
in their lives.

Sometimes I just say thank you to each ingredient:

Thank you, carrots. Thank you, potatoes.

Thank you, rice. Thank you, Mr. or Ms. Salmon.

FINAL WORDS

**In the act of giving thanks, we become aware of the bless-
ings that are woven into our life.**

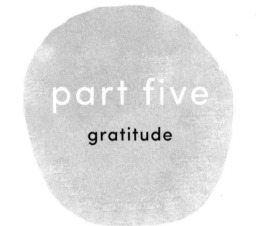

part five

gratitude

Without realizing it, we take so much for granted. This happens because our mind is not concerned with things that work well, like the earth continually growing our food, or the sun always appearing over the horizon at dawn, or hot water flowing out of the faucet when we turn it on, or not having a fever and cough. It is not until we are deprived of these ordinary things that we realize what blessings have been continually bestowed upon us.

Gratitude is the recognition that we have been given many gifts, not through our own actions but through the generosity of other people and also nonhuman sources such as animals, the rain, the earth, or God. The gifts can be material (clean water for bathing and drinking) or nonmaterial (emotional support). My first Zen teacher used to say, "When people tell me that they are overwhelmed with gratitude, I know that their meditation practice is working." When the heart and mind begin to settle and open, people start to appreciate that their life is composed not of an ongoing series of difficulties but of a continual flow of gifts.

Research shows that people who do a simple practice, writing down several things they are grateful for at the end of the day, have an increase in positive mood, satisfaction with life, optimism about the coming week, feelings of connection with others, and even the quality of their sleep.

The theologian Dietrich Bonhoeffer wrote, "In ordinary life we hardly realize that we receive a great deal more than we give, and that it is only with gratitude that life becomes rich."

21

gratitude
toward the body

the exercise

At least once a day, do a body scan with gratitude (described below). One convenient time is just after you lie down in bed at night. Another is during your usual time for meditation.

reminding yourself

Put a note on your bed pillow or on your meditation cushion saying "body scan with gratitude."

discoveries

Here is the exercise. See what *you* discover as you do it. In this meditation, we start from one end of the body, either the top of the head or the tips of the toes, moving our awareness sequentially through each body part. Our mind is used like a flashlight beam, a light we can direct toward one area at a time. As we focus on a part, we open our awareness to all the sensations arising in that part, including:

- temperature (the spectrum from warm to cold)

- touch (the many touches on the skin and inside the body, from barely to very noticeable)

- pressure (from light to very firm or even uncomfortable)

- movement (a linked series of touch sensations)

After you have focused your awareness on a body part, and just before moving on to the next part, say silently, "Thank you, [body part] for [fill in the blank]." Let whatever arises in the mind fill in the second blank. If nothing arises, that's fine.

If, for example, you have focused awareness on the chest and lungs, you become aware of all the sensations coming from the area of the chest and lungs. You are aware of these sensations as they arise, persist, and then fade away. Rest your awareness here as long as you like. Before moving on to another body part say silently, "Thank you, lungs for . . ." and allow a little gap. See if anything arises in that gap. If nothing comes up, that's OK too. Let's say what arises is "for breathing for me all these years, even at night when I'm asleep." Then move your mind's awareness on to another body part, perhaps the heart. As you repeat this meditation, try including body parts that you missed in earlier sessions. These might be internal organs such as the bladder or small parts such as eyelashes.

Pay special attention to body parts for which you detect some negative feelings. Include parts you don't like, such as wrinkles, abdominal fat, or a big nose. Include body parts that are having difficulties.

It is common for people who do this exercise to discover that they are irritated at body parts that they don't like (my teeth are crooked) or parts that are not functioning perfectly (why do my stupid lungs have asthma?). We may not be aware of our irritation or anger, but the body is aware of it. If an illness or disability lasts awhile or becomes chronic, then we can be bathing our body continually in the negative energy of our distress. An atmosphere of love and kindness is essential if living beings, including children, pets, plants, and our own bodies, are to thrive and reach their highest potential. When various parts of our body are in trouble, they need extra help and extra kindness, not extra criticism.

deeper lessons

When we are sick, the mind often says, "What's wrong with me? Why did I get sick?" The answer is, nothing is wrong. Your body being sick simply means that you are a being with a body. It is easy to become upset with our body when we have a cold, or constipation, diabetes, high blood pressure, painful joints, or when we just gain weight. We feel that our body has betrayed us.

Far from failing us, the body actually does an astounding job. Billions of cells in dozens of organs work continually, night and day, without pausing or taking a rest, for the entirety of our life. Thought is energy, and negative thoughts ("I hate my pudgy thighs," "I hate having a sore throat") have a negative effect. All living things wither under the energy of irritation and anger. All living things prosper under the warmth of gratitude and loving-kindness.

Most of us take our bodies and our good health for granted. In fact, we don't actually experience ourselves as "healthy" until we fall ill. If we've been sick in bed with a bad cold or the flu, too weak to get up or too nauseated to eat, it seems like a miracle when we begin to recover. For a few days it feels wondrous just to walk upright, to have an appetite, and to enjoy the smells and tastes of food again. If we've been in severe pain and it lifts, it can make us euphoric. Very soon, however, we go back to expecting our body to function well, to do what we ask it to do, efficiently and without discomfort.

When someone our own age becomes seriously ill or dies, it lifts the veil of denial, opening our eyes to the impermanence of health and life. We see clearly that health and life are temporary gifts. But we soon forget it again. When we forget, we fall back into irritation at our body. Why is my hearing going bad? Why does my back hurt? Why do I have allergies when other people don't? Why is my skin getting wrinkled so soon? How could I have gained weight?

Evolution designed our bodies to live thirty-five to forty years, long enough to reproduce and raise our young so they could survive on their own. After that age, we have outlived the warrantee on our body parts. Rationally we know that it is inevitable that our body will sometimes struggle and we will become ill. However, we still easily become critical toward it as it ages.

Mindful eating can help us bring awareness into our body, to feel and hear its messages from the inside, and then to direct the positive energy of gratitude and loving-kindness toward it. These meditations have the added benefit of helping us tune in to the signals of cellular hunger and also to the body's signals of satiation and satisfaction.

FINAL WORDS

Bathe your body regularly in gratitude and loving-kindness.
It will help it thrive.

looking deeply
into your food

the exercise

At least once a day, as you sit down to eat, pick out one piece of food from your meal—perhaps a carrot, a piece of lettuce, or a slice of bread—and do the exercise below, looking deeply into its history and the people and other beings who brought it to you.

reminding yourself

Post a note saying "look deeply" or a picture of eyes with beams coming out of them in places where you usually eat.

discoveries

Notice colors, shades, shapes, surface texture. This is the way we nourish ourselves through the eyes. However, there is another way of looking while eating—looking deeply into our food. This looking involves a different sense than our ordinary eyes: the inner eye. Imagine that you can see into the history of this bit of food. It is like seeing a movie of the food's life, but it is running backward. You keep asking, "And before that?" I'll use the example of the pieces of carrot in your soup.

You see how the carrots came to your bowl. Before that you might see them in the kitchen. You see the person who chopped and cooked the carrot. Before that you see the person who bought the carrots and brought them home and put them in the refrigerator. Before that you see the store, and you see the checkout clerk scanning the bag of carrots, and before that the produce staff who arranged the carrots in a display. Before that there was the person who unloaded the big boxes of carrots, and before that the delivery truck driver.

Now you take over, asking who came before the truck driver? Keep going backward, looking with the inner eye at all the living beings—people, animals, and plants—whose life energy flowed into this carrot and brought it to your soup. When you reach the carrot plant, ask where it came from and continue to extend your vision backward in time. Go as far back as you can.

Now we ask some questions:

- How many people were involved in bringing this piece of carrot to you?

- If you include all the animals, plants, insects, worms, and microscopic organisms that had a role in the life of this carrot, how many forms of life have contributed their life energy to bringing the carrot to you?

Invite all these people and other beings to gather around you in your imagination. As you eat mindfully, thank them all.

If you find your mind wandering to the injustices of factory farming or poor treatment of farm workers, consider this, "What can I do *right now*, as I eat this food, to recognize this gift?" You can give thanks for the lives that enable your life. Then if you wish, tomorrow you can get to work for better treatment of animals or farm laborers.

deeper lessons

At our Zen monastery, we chant short verses, or *gathas*, before meals. One of them is "Seventy-two labors brought us this food. We should know how it comes to us." (Traditionally there are seventy-two jobs that must be done to maintain a monastery, to keep it open and available to all.) This reminds us, no matter how hungry we are, to pause before eating and reflect upon the life energy that went into bringing the food to the table before us.

Through mindfulness, we can look more deeply into everyday things. It is a part of wisdom not to be fooled by the superficial aspects of things, even of the most ordinary things that we encounter many times a day. Food is one of these.

When we look deeply into our food, we find ourselves in the company of many beings whose life energy is a part of what we are about to eat. According to the Zen teachings, each time we eat, we take the life energy of countless beings into our bodies. The food on our plate is the product of the sun, the earth, the rain, the insects who pollinate the plants, and people of many sizes, shapes, ages, and nationalities, including farmers, captain and crew on a boat, truck drivers, and grocers.

This energy, which is the product of so many beings, courses through our body, propelled by every beat of our heart. It travels to the farthest cells, to our toenails and to the tips of our hair. The life energy of all these beings literally becomes us, our blue or brown eyes, our soft lips, our hard white teeth, our loving heart. This daily miracle of transubstantiation occurs in our own bodies, day and night.

Unfortunately, while this miracle is occurring we are mostly unaware of it. To awaken to it, even for a few moments each day, can give us new joy, no matter how difficult the other circumstances of our life may be. It can give us new energy, regardless of our age or how tired we are. If we eat with our mind open and aware, we can experience our intimate connection to these many beings, and our loneliness dissolves.

FINAL WORDS

The life energy of many beings flows into us as we eat and drink. How can we best thank them? By eating with awareness—and gratitude.

part six

mindful eating
with others

When we are first relearning how to be present as we eat, we need the support of a quiet environment, without distractions. We may need to close the office door while we eat lunch. We may need to step outside and sit on the step or a porch chair as we sip a hot drink. We may need a little more time in the beginning in order to slow down and be fully immersed in the smells, colors, textures, and flavors of eating.

But because this is something we once knew in our infancy—to simply eat, enjoy food, and to stop when full—we are able to pick up these old skills again fairly rapidly. Then we are able to eat quickly—when needed—with full awareness of both flavor and fullness and even awareness of the cells' responses to what we are eating. Because it is much more interesting to be present than to be spaced out, to be curious than to be bored, we begin to look forward to what we might discover at the next meal.

When we've learned to purposely pay attention when we're eating alone, the next step is to bring those skills into the world of other people—office lunchrooms, eating out with friends, and family meals. Here's how to accomplish that.

23

alternating practice

the exercise

When you are eating and talking with others, try alternating where you place the majority of your attention:
outward, into the conversation; or inward, into your mouth,
stomach, and body.

reminding yourself

Post a note saying "alternating practice" in your lunch box
or places where you usually eat with others.

discoveries

The most common question people ask when they begin
to learn mindful eating is, "I'm able to be attentive when
I'm alone and I can focus, but how can I do it when I'm
with my family or friends and they want to talk?" The
answer is a skill called "alternating practice."

It is much easier to practice mindful eating at first when there are no distractions. You can take the time to assess the Nine Hungers before you start eating, notice when your mind wanders off, and then bring it back to your mouth and body, keeping track of how full your stomach is becoming. You can stop to assess the hungers again before deciding whether to take seconds, and again after eating, to see if you estimated the right amount.

The difficulties arise when you try to practice mindful eating while having a normal conversation with family or friends. This is a real dilemma. It is impossible to pay 100 percent attention to two things at once. You can try it right now.

Put your full attention in your left big toe. Hold it there for a few seconds. Now move your attention to your right ear lobe. Hold it there. Now pay full attention to both your left big toe and your right ear lobe. What happens?

Most people find that their mind vacillates back and forth—toe, ear lobe, toe, ear lobe. That vacillation is exactly the key to being able to practice mindful eating while in the company of others. You will need to purposely switch the majority of your attention back and forth, between what is in your mouth and listening to the conversation. You will end up doing a lot more listening than talking: both "listening" to your inner companions—your mouth, stomach, and body—and also listening more carefully to your outer companions.

With alternating practice, when you have food in your mouth, most of your attention is in your mouth, but some is on what others are saying. After you swallow and your mouth is empty, you switch and bring most of your attention to the conversation. Once you've learned how to bring awareness to the nine aspects of hunger, alternating practice is a skill you can learn fairly quickly.

deeper lessons

Another way to make it easier to practice mindful eating in company is to enlist their help. When you are with others, let them know that you are trying to relax and be present as you eat. Or that you are trying to change the way you eat by doing this new thing called mindful eating. Ask them to help you with a few minutes of silence at the start of the meal so you can really appreciate the food. It's difficult for people to refuse a sincere request for support. Assess the Nine Hungers and savor the first tastes. When a new dish or dessert arrives, do this again. ("I would like to stop talking for a few seconds so I can really pay attention to the flavors of this delicious-looking dessert.") You can make a cook very happy when you truly enjoy the food they have prepared.

North Americans tend to be very independent and self-sufficient. It's hard for us to ask for help. But asking for help can open doors. It enables others to be generous and to become interested in new ideas and ways of being that you are exploring in your life. It also can help the conversation move more swiftly past the usual superficial chatter and into more nourishing content.

Alternating practice is a key component of living mindfully. We pay full attention to the next bite of food, and then we put down our fork and put full attention on answering an e-mail. We pay full attention to driving, and then we pull over and stop when we need to pay full attention to texting or talking on the phone. If we are reading a book, we close it and turn our eyes to our partner when they want to talk. In a complex, fast-paced life it is tempting to multitask, to eat while driving to our next appointment, to gulp our coffee mindlessly while reading a report, to keep on typing on the computer while talking to our kids. It's not that we never multitask or never eat mindlessly. Life sometimes makes it necessary, but we try to do it consciously, with awareness. In other words, mindful eating includes mindless eating, but we are aware that we are eating mindlessly. "Now I am doing three things at once. I am talking on the phone and sipping coffee, and I have one ear open to whether the baby has awakened."

"There's an urgent e-mail so I am answering it while eating lunch at my desk."

Realizing that we are eating mindlessly is the key. Awareness is the key. Once we are aware, we have a choice. Shall I do alternating practice? Can I stop eating for a few minutes in order to write the e-mail, then turn my attention away from the computer and eat a few bites with full awareness? Or am I in such a rush that I have to eat and write at the same time? If I'm in an unavoidable rush now, I can promise myself the treat of eating supper tonight undistracted.

FINAL WORDS

Mindful eating can include mindless eating, but we are aware that we are eating mindlessly. Remember that alternating practice is always an option.

summary tips

In this book we've explored a great deal of information and quite a few practices. Here's a quick review of the essential points. It might be helpful to return to this list from time to time, as you work to make mindful eating a part of your everyday life.

- Mindful eating is about opening the mind's awareness to our food and to the body, before, during, and after we eat.

- Mindful eating is nonjudgmental.

- Awareness is the key to change. Once we are aware of something, it cannot remain the same. Awareness plus small changes in our automatic behaviors can produce large changes over time. Awareness means choice and choice means freedom.

- Learn to assess stomach and cellular hunger before you eat, during eating, and after eating.

- Practice all Nine Hungers until you can do it fairly quickly.

- If you are not hungry, don't eat.

- Be present for at least the first three bites or sips as you begin to eat or drink.

- At least once a week, eat an entire meal in silence and mindfulness.

- Eat small portions, considering the "right amount." For your first helping, serve yourself an amount of food that will leave you two-thirds full.

- Eat slowly, savoring each bite. Find ways of pausing as you eat, such as putting down your fork or spoon between bites.

- Chew your food thoroughly before swallowing.

- Become aware of the difference between "no longer hungry" and "full." There is no need to eat all the way to full. Eat until you are 80 percent full, then take a drink and rest a bit.

- Mindful eating sometimes includes mindless eating. You can choose to eat mindlessly when it is appropriate.

- Emptying is as important as filling. This applies both to the stomach and to the mind.

- Know that food changes mood and use it as good medicine. Adjust the dose; if you eat mindfully, a small amount may work better than a lot.

- Above all, know when it is not the body but the heart that is asking to be fed. Give it the nutrition that fills it up. That nutrition could be meditation or prayer, walking, being in nature, listening to or making music, playing with a pet, fixing food for someone you love or who needs help, or just sitting and being present with people.

- Remember, a hole in the heart cannot be filled with food. Fill the heart with the richness of this very moment.

- Before, during, and after eating, give thanks.

list of audio tracks

This book is accompanied with audio tracks of guided meditations and other exercises to assist you in your mindfulness practice, available at www.shambhala.com /mindfuleating.

1. Introduction

2. The Basic Mindful Eating Meditation

3. Asking the Body What It Needs

4. Who Is Hungry in There? Examining the Nine Hungers

5. Food and Mood

6. Slow It Down (Put Down That Fork and Spoon)

7. Taking in the Right Amount

8. Basic Meditation Instructions

9. Loving-Kindness toward the Body

about the author

Jan Chozen Bays, MD, is a pediatrician, Zen teacher, wife, mother, and grandmother. She has studied and practiced Zen since 1973 and has taught mindful eating for more than three decades to individuals and healthcare professionals. Dr. Bays worked for thirty years at Legacy Children's Hospital in Portland, Oregon. She received her Zen training under the revered Zen master Taizan Maezumi Roshi and then under Shodo Harada Roshi, abbot of Sogen-ji monastery in Japan. She is the coabbot of the Great Vow Zen Monastery in Clatskanie, Oregon, and the author of *Jizo Bodhisattva, How to Train a Wild Elephant, Mindfulness on the Go,* and *The Vow-Powered Life*. She loves to garden, bake bread, play marimba, and square dance.

For more information, visit www.zendust.org/about /mindful-eating.